'In a world of ever increasing pressure and pace, Nora's traditional wisdom provides a rare place of calm reflection and insight. I love her ability to distil simplicity from complexity and clarity from opacity. That so much of her writing is based on observing everyday life, and lightly drawing the deeper meanings from it, is what makes the work so accessible and all the more precious.'

*— Jeremy Sweeney, Executive Coach, London*

'I return to Nora's blog again and again for her insights into the human condition. I feel as though I'm part of a conversation in which I'm enlightened, reassured and uplifted. Nora has a knack of getting to the heart of the matter by explaining profound and complicated ideas simply and easily. Her blogs are always thought provoking and life-affirming.'

*— Susan Vale, designer, Hampshire*

'Nora writes with such joy from her heart that you feel her warmth, humour and wisdom in every blog post. Her deep understanding of the five elements and her intricate observations of life and people trigger your senses and ignite your imagination.'

*— Jian Ling Shen, Mandarin teacher, London*

# BLOGGING
## A FIVE
# ELEMENT LIFE

*by the same author*

**On Being a Five Element Acupuncturist**
ISBN 978 1 84819 236 2
eISBN 978 0 85701 183 1
Part of the Five Element Acupuncture series

**The Handbook of Five Element Practice**
ISBN 978 1 84819 188 4
eISBN 978 0 85701 145 9
Part of the Five Element Acupuncture series

**Patterns of Practice**
**Mastering the Art of Five Element Acupuncture**
ISBN 978 1 84819 187 7
eISBN 978 0 85701 148 0
Part of the Five Element Acupuncture series

**Keepers of the Soul**
**The Five Guardian Elements of Acupuncture**
ISBN 978 1 84819 185 3
eISBN 978 0 85701 146 6
Part of the Five Element Acupuncture series

**The Simple Guide to Five Element Acupuncture**
ISBN 978 1 84819 186 0
eISBN 978 0 85701 147 3
Part of the Five Element Acupuncture series

# BLOGGING
# A FIVE
# ELEMENT LIFE

NORA FRANGLEN

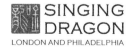

SINGING
DRAGON
LONDON AND PHILADELPHIA

First published in 2017
by Singing Dragon
an imprint of Jessica Kingsley Publishers
73 Collier Street
London N1 9BE, UK
and
400 Market Street, Suite 400
Philadelphia, PA 19106, USA

*www.singingdragon.com*

Copyright © Nora Franglen 2017

Front cover image source: StockSnap®.

**Library of Congress Cataloging in Publication Data**
A CIP catalog record for this book is available from the Library of Congress

**British Library Cataloguing in Publication Data**
A CIP catalogue record for this book is available from the British Library

ISBN 978 1 84819 371 0
eISBN 978 0 85701 328 6

Printed and bound by CPI Group (UK) Ltd, Croydon, CR0 4YY

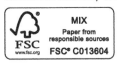

MIX
Paper from
responsible sources
FSC
www.fsc.org
FSC® C013604

*For my family*

# CONTENTS

# INTRODUCTION

This is my second book of blogs. My first, *On Being a Five Element Acupuncturist*, covered the period from 2010 to 2013. This book continues on from then, ending in March 2017.

I often ask myself why I so much enjoy writing blogs, and I think it is because I love passing my thoughts on. Each blog is a communication between me and whoever is out there reading them. I don't write them because I want feedback from my readers, and the same holds true for my other writing, that of my books. The important thing for me is that my thoughts should be sent out into the world, and, as I love words, in the form of words.

I regard each blog therefore as representing a thought, something which has occurred to me, often sparked by the thoughts of others, such as in books I read or conversations I have. If I worked in a visual medium, a blog would then be like a painting, encapsulating one moment in time, whilst my books would be more like a film extending over time.

Whenever I write, I like to think about something a very wise old Viennese musician and astrologer, Dr Oskar Adler, a friend of my family, wrote in one of his books. He said, 'Everybody has a duty to pass on whatever they have learnt. You never know who will read it and who will learn from it.'

Since I started writing, in my late 40s, quite late in my life, I hear his words echoing in my mind. So each blog I write, each representing a thought of mine, is my acknowledgement of what Dr Adler said. For who know where these snippets of thoughts of mine are ending up? I will never know, but I like to think of them winging their way through the ether in blog form or over the seas in book form, as here, for the many people round the world who sign up to read my blog.

◇◇◇◇◇◇◇◇◇◇◇◇◇◇ 2014 BLOGS ◇◇◇◇◇◇◇◇◇◇◇◇◇◇

# 1 JANUARY 2014

## *The importance of getting feedback from other practitioners*

Because it is so difficult to pinpoint one element out of the five which stamps a person's life with their individuality, we can be guilty of trying to simplify things by sticking to rather rigid guidelines by which we judge the elements. This can become a kind of false short-cut without our being aware of this, and we can then refuse to deviate from these whatever the evidence which should be persuading us to modify our understanding. We should never say things like 'Oh, this is obviously Wood' or 'It can only be Earth.' We should always say, 'I think this is…' and wait for time and good treatment to confirm or alter our opinion.

I can still remember my amazement that a patient I was absolutely sure was Fire turned out instead to be Metal when this was pointed out by a tutor. And I only really began to understand the Earth element's need to turn thoughts over and over in their mind when a patient of mine I was sure was Fire proved instead to be an excellent example of Earth. In both cases, I had to stop myself from expressing my initial reaction, which was 'Oh, no, I think you're wrong', forcing myself instead to face the fact that I still had so much to learn.

So any five element acupuncturist reading this should take what I am writing to heart. We always need those with more experience than we have to open our eyes (and ears and noses!) to deeper levels of understanding. Even now, after more than 30 years of studying the elements, they continue to surprise me with some unexpected display of an aspect I did not associate with them. Good five element acupuncturists must never mind stumbling around for a time in the unknown, because every new person we meet is an unknown.

It's what makes our work so exciting. That is, of course, one of the delights, to me, of my practice. Thank goodness it will always be challenging, never boring.

◇◇◇◇◇◇◇◇

# 1 JANUARY 2014
## *Translating my blogs into Mandarin*

As I have blogged before, I am planning to publish my blogs of the past three years (or a significant selection of them) in book form in the New Year, if Singing Dragon is happy to add a fifth book of mine to the four they have just republished (see my blog for 18 November 2013). I regard these blogs, specifically those about my acupuncture practice, as an essential component of my teaching work, and therefore of particular relevance to my Chinese students. Mei has already translated parts of my blog to add to the mini-blog she sends regularly to China, but this has so far been on a very ad-hoc basis, depending on the time she has available.

I now think it is time to make sure that anything I write which I think will be particularly useful for my Chinese students to learn from should be translated into Mandarin on a regular basis, rather than in the somewhat haphazard way that now happens.

As things happen, or as they seem constantly to happen to me in relation to my Chinese adventures, an opportunity has now presented itself to do just this. A very enthusiastic Chinese acupuncturist from Chengdu, Caroline, who has an excellent understanding of English, has volunteered to translate my blogs as I write them. So I hope today's blog, which is now speeding through the ether to China, will become the first in this new regular publication of my thoughts for a Chinese audience.

Thank you, Caroline, for offering to help all those who can only read my blogs in Mandarin.

And a very Happy New Year to all my readers!

◇◇◇◇◇◇◇◇◇

# 1 JANUARY 2014
## *How much do we owe our patients?*

I asked this question of myself just before Christmas when a long-term patient of mine unexpectedly appeared after quite a long absence abroad and expected a treatment at the start of my Christmas holiday period, almost, I felt, as though by right. In the past I think I would have felt compelled to make every effort to fit him in, even though I was officially already on holiday, and I did a lot of heart-searching along the lines of 'Why did he not have the good sense (and courtesy) to get in touch beforehand to check whether I would be available?'

At the start of his treatment, many years ago, we had done a lot of good work together, and he attributed the regaining of his good health entirely to his acupuncture treatment. This long and successful association made me feel very close to him, and has in the past persuaded me to make every effort to fit him in on his infrequent and very brief visits to London from abroad. But when I heard his voice on the answering machine, I realized that, with my new-found aim of looking after myself a little more and not placing myself under too much stress, a good Christmas break was more important for my well-being, rather than readjusting my schedule to fit him in at the last minute, as I used to do. So I didn't treat him, but suggested he contact a colleague of mine, which he decided not to do.

Each practitioner has to work out the parameters within which he/she works. Mine, I realize, have not been as rigid and as carefully delineated as I have told my students they should be. In other words, I am often a bit of a pushover for patients in need.

Perhaps this recent example is a sign that I am at last learning to harden my heart a little more than I have done in the past.

◇◇◇◇◇◇◇◇◇

# 2 JANUARY 2014
## *English translation of the wording on the back cover of* Les gardiens de l'âme, *the French edition of my* Keepers of the Soul

Sylviane Burner, the excellent translator of my *Keepers of the Soul, Les gardiens de l'âme*, now published by Satas of Belgium (www.satas.com), has written a very moving tribute to my book which appears on its back cover. I have in turn translated this into English, and have her permission to reproduce it below. She has a true feeling for what my book is about, and I am privileged to have her as translator of what is definitely my most complex book.

> *The Keepers of the Soul: The Five Guardian Elements of Acupuncture* by Nora Franglen is not simply another book about acupuncture. The author does, of course,

talk about acupuncture, discussing the mysterious qualities of the five elements (Wood, Fire, Earth, Metal and Water), which she has studied in depth as a five element acupuncturist. Starting with the correspondences between the elements and nature and the seasons, she writes about each of them in detail and with a rare poetical approach. Taking the reader on a journey of initiation into great universal truths and into the most intimate depths of ourselves, we are told about the characteristics, strengths and weaknesses which our guardian element, our constitutional element, has bestowed upon us since our birth. Acupuncturists will learn to use the five elements, and most particularly our guardian element, to correct the imbalances we suffer from, and psychologists will discover the subtle workings of this guardian element which places its seal upon the personality of each one of us; with surprise, we will learn to understand why we react as we do, why we behave as we do, why we are attracted to some people as we are, why we are frightened by what we are – in other words, what makes us who we are as individuals. Step by step, subtly and gently, and with enthusiasm and humility, Nora Franglen guides us through the complexities and byways of the human soul, truly a voyage into the infinite which opens up for us many perspectives to help us relate more easily to ourselves and to others, and to understand why, faced with the same situation, each of us will react either in the same or a quite different way. In this journey into ourselves, as we pass through the cycle of the seasons at the whim of the vagaries of life, accompanied by an element which emphasizes our relationship to these seasons, it is our guardian element, truly a keeper of the soul, which will guide us throughout our life.

*Sylviane Burner*

◇◇◇◇◇◇◇◇

# 10 JANUARY 2014
## *A happy day, or what a simple smile can do*

There was no particular reason why today became such a happy day for me, except perhaps for the fact that the sun was shining, dispelling the wind and the rain of the dreadful last few days of storm and tempest. I suppose that was reason enough, though, for me to smile, and I realize after a day of exchanging smiles with everybody I came in contact with that when you smile the world smiles with you.

So as I moved from bus to greengrocer, to library, to bookshop, interspersed with a series of coffee bars (my usual daily haunts), a gentle layer of joy was laid over my day. It even gifted me with the unexpected bonus of a lunchtime concert at St James's Piccadilly, as I passed through the church and heard an excellent pianist practising works I had never heard before but which delighted me.

Now it has started to rain again, but I hope that the rain will not wipe the smile from my face.

◇◇◇◇◇◇◇◇

# 10 JANUARY 2014
## *Approach to treating a very ill patient*

Learning to cope with treating very ill patients has always been one of the hardest things for me to do, as it probably is for practitioners of any medical discipline. This is made even more difficult when I am asked to treat a long-standing patient with whom I have built up a close relationship over the years. This has now happened in the case of one of my patients.

This patient has been fighting a complex history of severe ill-health over many years, and to the surprise of many has managed to stay as healthy as she has through what she maintains is help not only from her Western medical team but from her regular acupuncture treatments. The chance that she would continue to live as productive a life as she has over the past few years must already have been rather slim, but I always lived in hope that what I was doing with the needle might be miraculous enough to stave off more serious illness. Sadly, this has not been the case, and she is back in hospital on a morphine drip, and has asked me to come and treat her there. I have now visited her twice, and at each visit I am faced with having to decide what treatment to give.

We all have a tendency to blame our own inadequacy when a patient succumbs to ill-health, so I had first to remind myself not to regard what I had done so far as a failure. I had to tell myself that I had done the best I could. Looking at the notes I made the last time she came for a treatment a few weeks ago, I see that she told me that everything in her life was going well and she was feeling fine. We were then neither of us to know that this illness would descend upon her so suddenly like a tragic bolt from the blue.

It is always difficult treating somebody in hospital. We can't use moxa because of the risk of setting off the fire alarms, and access to a patient in a hospital bed, attached to various drips, is always somewhat hazardous, and requires us to move carefully round the bed, manoeuvring ourselves past the apparatus and the bedside table with all its necessary paraphernalia. Then we have to consider how far it is fair to ask an already uncomfortable patient to change position or to sit up to expose the back. Bl 38 (43), that most wondrous point which 'helps every cell in the body', as JR Worsley told us, is therefore sometimes ruled out altogether, or is difficult to locate when perhaps only a small area of the back is available to us and finding the scapula proves difficult. Certainly the many moxa cones it needs to do its miraculous work are unfortunately out of the question. Luckily, at my last visit, my patient's husband appeared at just the right moment to help prop his wife up slightly to expose the top of the back. But I still had to send a prayer up to heaven asking for help in locating the point, so little of the back could I see. There was no question of doing an Aggressive Energy (AE) drain at either visit, as I would have liked to have done.

Then, because her lungs were very painful and her breathing laboured, I decided I needed to clear what I assumed to be an VIII/IX (Liver/Lung) Entry/Exit block, even though my pulse-readings did not absolutely confirm this for me, pulses also being difficult to take and to interpret in view of all the medication she is being given. Again, I could hardly find the ribs because of a distended stomach, and hoped that I correctly needled Liv 14, and not some other point on the abdomen. Lu 1 was much easier to find, and I finished the treatment with command points on the Water element, her guardian element. As I left, I was delighted to receive confirmation that I had indeed got the points when she suddenly said, with surprise in her voice, 'I really feel better.' How long this improvement will last only time will tell, but evidence of even the slightest relief was a gift to me, and sent me home slightly happier, as I left her sleeping peacefully, her breathing less laboured.

I'm not sure which of the points I needled helped her feel better, or whether it was a combination of all of them. I like to think that it is probably clearing the Liver/Lung block which had the biggest effect, but it really doesn't matter and I will never know. The important thing is that, as I left, she had a slight smile on her face which lightened my journey home.

At my first visit last week, she was lying in such a position that I was able only to reach the source points of Water on her feet, but again these were effective, removing that desperate look in the eyes which very ill patients have. I interpreted the change in her to her Water element regaining control of her fear. This look of fear had not returned when I saw her the second time, even though her physical condition had deteriorated.

The prognosis is not good, but I will continue to do whatever I can to help the elements ease her pain and distress.

◇◇◇◇◇◇◇◇◇

# 16 JANUARY 2016
## *Chinese blog for my Mandarin blog translations*

Caroline, a five element practitioner from Chengdu (see my blog of 1 January 2014), has now set up a special blog in China to which she will post her translations of this blog. So now I will go through my recent blogs and send her any which I feel will be helpful for my Chinese students.

Oh, the wonders of modern technology never fail to impress me (and depress me, too, if I can't work my way round them, as I often can't).

◇◇◇◇◇◇◇◇

## 4 FEBRUARY 2014
### *My third hospital visit to treat my patient*

I never know whether what I am doing helps my patients until they themselves provide me with evidence of improvement. Assessing the result of a previous treatment in the case of a very ill patient therefore becomes all the more crucial. This week I was blessed with hearing my patient say as I approached her hospital bed, 'Nora, they are amazed at how well I am.' And I was amazed, too. She is still having weekly chemotherapy, and is tolerating the side-effects surprisingly well. She is still on painkillers, but no longer needs morphine, and her lungs are now functioning without distressing her so that she has no need of additional oxygen.

Her eyes were bright, and she was surprisingly cheerful, considering that she is suffering from painful bedsores. They are thinking of allowing her home in a few weeks once she has completed the chemotherapy sessions. The hospital can't believe that she is tolerating the chemotherapy so well, but I know that Bl 38 (43), that miracle point for helping the blood, can indeed produce miracles and help her body cope as well as it is with the poisons being pumped into it.

My treatment this time was Bl 38 again (one of the few points in five element acupuncture which can be used repeatedly), IV (Ki) 16, which JR Worsley told us is like a

III 38 of the Kidney, finishing with III (Bl) 67 and IV (Ki) 7, the tonification points.

I will see her again in a week and hope that the improvement continues. As I left, she called out to me, 'I love you,' which sent me on my way with tears in my eyes.

I wish, though, that I could have used the moxa stick to help her bedsores, but the smoke would not be allowed because it might set off the fire alarms. One of my patients managed to persuade the doctors to let her sister use it on her bedsores in hospital, and told me that they cleared up miraculously quickly. If I were younger, I would like to have looked at doing some research on the moxa stick and its ability to help all kinds of skin problems. Often, bedsores for the bedridden are the most painful thing they have to suffer, and could so easily be helped with this little magical stick of mugwort, the support of the medical staff and a little bit of inventiveness at finding a place with some suitable outside ventilation.

◇◇◇◇◇◇◇◇

# 9 FEBRUARY 2014
## *The moxa stick*

I have been asked to describe how the moxa stick (a cigar-shaped roll of mugwort, encased in paper) can be used to help bedsores (see my last blog). In order not to reinvent the wheel, I am attaching below a handout I gave my students at the School of Five Element Acupuncture (SOFEA) some years ago which covers all the points I would like to make now. It's rather a long handout, because there are so many uses to which we can put the moxa stick!

Mugwort appears to help cell regeneration and heals at a very deep level. Its heat, if applied for a sufficiently long time over traumatized tissue, will eventually draw blood to the surface, and the action of blood helps in numerous ways to restore the body to health. Everybody should be encouraged to have a moxa stick at home because it is one of the most effective ways of dispelling pain, getting rid of infection and general healing that I know of. For non-acupuncturists reading this, you can buy moxa sticks from any acupuncture supplier. It's also sensible to buy a moxa stick holder at the same time to help extinguish the stick at the end of use, though a suitable-sized candlestick is just as good.

I give below some of the many successful uses of moxa from my own practice. In many cases the moxa stick was used as a support to acupuncture treatment, but it is very effective on its own.

**How to use it**

You don't need to remove the paper covering, a common failing with those using it for the first time. This holds the moxa in place. The stick can be lit through the paper. It takes some time to light the stick properly, so be patient. A great deal of smoke must come from it and you must feel great heat from the tip before you start applying it. It often goes out, and has to be relit. To do this, cut off the few centimetres of ash before starting to relight it. You need a lot of patience using the stick, so you must prepare your patients for this. There is no point whatsoever applying lukewarm heat. The stick must be so hot that it becomes painful after a little time, at which point you draw the stick slightly further away,

*Action*

Move the stick slowly over the area to be healed, keeping it as close to the skin as possible so that it receives maximum heat.

Tell the patient to tell you when it gets too hot so that you can draw it away a little. It is important that maximum heat is applied, and that you warn the patient that it will get very hot, and that that is essential. Obviously, be careful not to blister the skin. Don't move the stick over too wide an area (an area of a few centimetres at a time is better), because the skin will cool down too quickly between applications. You need concentrated heat for the stick to work.

Obviously, it is easier if the patient applies the stick him/herself, as they are better able to control the heat, but this is only possible on areas of the skin which can be reached by them.

For any very localized problem, such as a small cut, do not move the stick at all, but hold it in one position as close to the skin as possible, withdrawing it only when it becomes too hot for the patient to tolerate. This draws the infection out of the area, and is particularly successful with things like boils or whiteheads. In these cases, you go as close to the skin as possible, wait until the patient tells you it is very hot and draw the stick away completely for a few seconds to allow the area to cool down a little, before reapplying.

*How often do you use the stick?*

There have to be frequent applications for any stubborn infection or skin condition to be relieved. These must be at least once a day, for a period of at least ten minutes and longer if the patient has the patience. The longer and the more frequent the better. One of my patients with very severe psoriasis over large areas of the body applied the stick for at least half an hour twice a day very successfully. It took about two weeks for the very bad patches to disappear. There is no contraindication to the frequency of use.

## What it can be used for

*Any infected area at all*

This means things like ulcers, such as those caused by bedsores, infected fingers, infected scar tissue or toothache caused by an infected tooth.

*Any skin complaints whatsoever*

Particularly stubborn ones like psoriasis. Psoriasis leaves a layer of dead skin on the surface, which eventually cracks and leads to bleeding below it. A patient should be given a supply of moxa sticks and told to use it over the most affected area of traumatized skin. Because the heat has to penetrate the dead skin, it will take some time for the patient to feel any warmth, and the application of the moxa stick must continue until the area to which it is being applied becomes really warm to the touch and remains warm once the stick is removed. Often the psoriasis is over a very wide area of the body, and it would take too long to moxa every patch of psoriasis. I have found, though, that really concentrating on one small patch has an effect throughout the body, as if the healing in one area leads to healing in another. So try one patch at a time. Since the patient will do most of the work (although you can help a little each time he/she comes for treatment), it is important that you don't give them too great a task to do; otherwise they won't do it. Time taken: Probably at least ten minutes on each badly infected patch until it glows with warmth.

You know things are moving if the dry skin starts to drop off, the bleeding stops and a layer of fresh new, pink skin appears round the edges of the psoriasis patches. This is the new skin forming below the surface which eventually pushes off the dead skin. Carry on moxaing over the new skin, but more gently and from further away, as it is very delicate and you obviously don't want to blister it.

If the skin complaint is on the face, such as pimples, where the moxa could burn the skin, place a layer of paper between the skin and the stick as protection, placing your hands carefully over the paper so that is does not get so hot as to burn. The skin should be red and glowing when you finish, so suggest the patient does the moxaing in the evening, not just before they go out to work.

*Boils*

For very localized skin complaints, such as boils, do not move the stick, but hold it straight over the boil. You will find that the infected material will gradually be drawn out to the surface through the heat.

*Whiteheads*

These can cause quite unsightly lumps on the skin, and are usually removed surgically. The method for removing them is to hold the stick closely above them. Again, the impacted sebaceous gland will heal itself, releasing the sebum. If it is a large whitehead, it may leave a little crater, possibly with some residual infection. If this is so, carry on moxaing until the area looks really healed.

*Cuts and blisters*

If there is bleeding, you can see a layer of healed tissue forming very soon after you moxa. Large and weeping blisters will disappear overnight if moxa is applied. Cuts also heal very much more quickly.

*Surgical adhesions*

If there is scarring either on or below the surface after surgery which is causing adhesions, applying the moxa stick over the area will help the distressed scar tissue reintegrate better. A patient of mine had had a hysterectomy two years before, and the scar still tugged painfully deep inside. She used the stick successfully to get rid of the pain. She said she could feel the tightness loosening as she applied the moxa stick. It is very important to give a patient recovering from any form of surgery a stick to speed the healing, and it is excellent to get rid of infections over the surgical area, for example in the case of a Caesarean.

### Viral complaints such as herpes and shingles

I suggested that one of my patients should use the stick on a painful herpes patch of skin on her buttock which appeared at the time of each period. To my surprise, it disappeared after one application, never to re-occur. I have also given it to a patient with shingles, and this alleviated the pain enormously. I imagine it would also help chickenpox sufferers but I have not yet had an opportunity to try this out.

### Pain of any kind

Wherever there is pain, such as aching joints, twisted ankles or soreness. The stick will help the area feel warm and loved, and the pain often goes or at least lessens.

### Drawing a splinter out

If you can't get the splinter out (i.e. if it is deeply below a nail), moxa over the nail. This will get rid of any infection that might build up under the nail, and I have found that the splinter is gradually pushed out as the nail grows.

Finally, the secret is always to think of the moxa stick if there is any problem on the surface of the skin. If the patient feels better from doing it, then tell him/her to carry on; if worse (which I have actually never found), then to stop. If nothing happens after 4–5 days of application, then there is no point continuing because it is ineffective.

**Three warnings**

1. Patients (and practitioners) often don't apply the heat for long enough or close enough to the skin. You have to get the technique right and have the patience and time to carry on applying the stick over some days for it to work.

2. Make sure you have extinguished the heated stick properly; otherwise it will continue to smoulder for a long time.

3. Because it creates quite a lot of smoke, it's best to use it in a well-ventilated room, or ideally outside in the open, such as in the garden. Some people find the smell it leaves behind quite strong, but don't allow that to stop you from using it!

I hope those reading this will start using the moxa stick more.

◇◇◇◇◇◇◇◇◇

# 16 FEBRUARY 2014
## *'The older mind may just be a fuller mind'*

It's heartening for somebody struggling as I am increasingly to remember the names of people, and assuming, like my contemporaries, that this is a sign of an aging mind, to read an article in *The Observer* today, quoting from another in *The New York Times*.

It appears that researchers in Germany are wondering whether indeed older minds may just be fuller minds, rather than atrophying minds. The article states, cheerily, 'Since educated older people generally know more words than younger people, the experiment simulates what an older brain has to do to retrieve a word. And when the researchers incorporated that difference into the models, most aging "deficits" disappeared.'

The article finishes on this happy note for me: 'It's not that you're slow. It's that you know so much.'

◇◇◇◇◇◇◇◇

## 18 FEBRUARY 2014
### *The wonders of the internet!*

Yesterday, out of the blue, I was amused to see that nearly 1000 people had suddenly signed on to read my blog, most of them looking at what I wrote about the moxa stick. Usually, the number is a sedate 50–100 a day.

When I traced this back, the majority of the page views had originated in Facebook accounts in the States. Somebody somewhere over there, who has a very active Facebook account, must have linked me in to their account by accident. There must be quite a few surprised Americans who have found themselves reading all about the uses of the moxa stick. And it's one of my longest blogs, too.

Today the number has dropped a little, but is well above 400, so some 600 of those viewing my blog yesterday have obviously felt no further urge to discover more about five element acupuncture. Acupuncture suppliers, though, may be surprised to find that orders for moxa sticks have increased substantially.

**Footnote to the above, added 22 February 2014**

All is now explained! My lovely publishers, Singing Dragon, shared my blog about the moxa stick (posted 9 February) on their Facebook page, www.facebook.com/SingingDragon, creating, as they put it, 'an enormous positive response'.

◇◇◇◇◇◇◇◇

# FEBRUARY 2014
## *A talk for the British Acupuncture Council at its Annual Conference in September 2014*

I have been asked to give the keynote address at the British Acupuncture Council's Annual Conference at the end of September 2014. I hesitated a little before accepting, since giving public talks is not what I wish to do now (except in China!), but then I decided to accept because what I have been asked to talk about is my role in the return of five element acupuncture to China. And that is something I feel very passionate about.

I have to provide a title for my talk, and two have so far occurred to me: *'Five element acupuncture comes full circle'* and *'The return of five element acupuncture to its roots in China'*. Probably I will decide on a title which brings these two thoughts together.

The real impetus to my accepting the BAC's invitation is my strong belief that everybody involved in acupuncture, particularly those practising what I call modern Chinese acupuncture, commonly known as TCM, should be aware of how little of the spirit is involved in its practice, whereas how much of the spirit there is in the classics which all Chinese acupuncturists still learn as though by rote. This leads to a kind of subtle schizophrenia in relation to their practice, where, my Chinese students tell me, no attention at all is paid to the spirit, despite it being so heavily emphasized in classical texts.

I feel the return of five element acupuncture to China is an important step towards bridging this unnecessary divide. And it is regarded as such by all I encounter in China. As one very senior regional official told me as I treated him, 'We have lost our soul in China. We need you here.'

◇◇◇◇◇◇◇◇◇

# 6 MARCH 2014
## *Encroaching upon the space of others*

I am more and more aware of how people appear to have less and less respect for the space of others. I am sure this must somehow be related to the increasing immersion in mobile phones as people walk around, which cocoons them in a private world. In the last few days I have noticed how often people walking towards me in the street, talking on their phones, or, worse still, texting with the undivided attention this requires, have often been so oblivious of my approach that they have bumped into me, or simply expected me to move out of the way. This is particularly noticeable when it rains, and umbrellas are added to the mix. I then not only have to take avoiding action but have to duck under the outstretched umbrellas of those so unaware of me.

With mobile phones, there is increasing interaction with people far away from us and increasingly less with those a mere few feet from us. This must surely impact upon human relationships, as it does upon the pleasure I take in a simple walk along the street.

◇◇◇◇◇◇◇◇◇

# 10 MARCH 2014
## *Today's dummy culture*

Why do all babies need dummies now? This question often occurs to me as I watch babies passing me on the street, all lustily sucking on dummies, or as I watch parents shove a dummy back into their offspring's mouth even when the baby is not crying out for it. Years ago, dummies were frowned upon; it was thought instead that if babies cried they should be given the warm nipple with its natural supply of comforting food rather than the unpleasant cold plastic variety which gives a baby nothing, however much the baby tries to suck from it.

I find it interesting to speculate why the dummy has become such a universal accessory to a baby's life. It worries me that babies now grow up being sold an illusion, tempted to believe, as the dummy goes in the mouth and stimulates the sucking reflex, that it will provide food, whilst it does nothing of the kind. It is a bit as though you offer somebody what appears to be a sweet in a lovely wrapping, only for them to find when the wrapping is undone that there is nothing inside after all. It can surely not be healthy to keep on disappointing a baby in this way.

It is little wonder, then, that so many people have problems relating to food in their later life, since all eating habits start in childhood, as we know. In five element terms, this shapes a person's relationship to their Earth element, the mother element. The provision of nourishment for her child, which is a mother's first task, should always be associated with the love and warmth of being held close to a mother, not the stuffing of a surrogate plastic nipple into a baby's mouth.

As I watch babies sucking feverishly on their dummies, my heart bleeds for what this is doing to the development of their Earth element, and their capacity to nourish themselves later in life. And perhaps, too, this goes some way to explain the sight of so many adults streaming along the road to work, all carrying their dummy-replacements, a plastic cup of coffee, as though they, too, have been brainwashed since childhood by the need to have something, anything, in their mouth to suck on.

Just as babies can't nowadays seem to do without a dummy, so adults can't seem to do without a cup of coffee in the hand.

◇◇◇◇◇◇◇◇

# 19 MARCH 2014
## *The stresses caused by inequality*

I am reading a very interesting book at the moment, *The Spirit Level: Why Equality is Better for Everyone* by Richard Wilkinson and Kate Pickett. It has made me think a lot about the particular stresses of modern life, and whether different countries are subject to different stresses. Since I am off to China again in a couple of weeks, it has become particularly relevant for me to look at what stresses we in this country are exposed to compared with those of the Chinese.

I am fascinated by the main message of the book which is how much extreme financial inequalities, such as those now experienced in this country, affect everybody, not just the poorest. I was interested to see, for example, that it was noticeable how local communities reacted in different ways in New Orleans in response to Hurricane Katrina in 2005, in contrast to the Chinese response to its devastating earthquake in 2008. In the much more settled local communities in China, there was much greater cooperation and help for the survivors than in New Orleans, with its very deprived communities, where looting and violence were the norm. Sadly, of course, as China, too, becomes an increasingly unequal society, with the rich now becoming the super-rich, the support of a local community is becoming as rare as in this country, where the rich are now holed up in their large houses behind barriers, and the poor hammer at the gates with rage.

All this increases the stresses of modern life in terms of mental health, alcoholism, obesity, infant mortality, the crime rate and much more, but equally affects those living behind those barred gates to a surprising degree. This is a terrible downward spiral, encapsulated for me in the headline yesterday in *The Guardian* newspaper which states baldly: 'Divided Britain: Five families own more than poorest 20%: Handful of super-rich are wealthier than 12.6m Britons put together'. Such enormous discrepancies in wealth, the authors of this book say, are the direct cause of some of the most complex types of modern illness, called, somewhat wittily, 'anxiety disorders', 'affluenza virus' or 'luxury fevers', as the status anxieties that a consumer society fosters in everybody cause increasing levels of stress, unknown by me as a child during and after the Second World War, when we didn't go shopping for evermore tantalizing goods because the shops were empty.

Nor did we feel the lack of this at all. I remember quite happily listening again and again to the few gramophone records we had, and reading again and again the few children's books we had, and not feeling deprived at all – rather the reverse.

The message obviously is that where there is satisfaction with our lives, whether we are poor or rich, the healthier and happier we will be. And the more status stress we cause ourselves by trying to emulate all the acquisitive habits of the rich (their clothes, their homes, their furnishings), the more illnesses we will suffer from. There is a lesson here for acupuncturists, since our aim must surely be to help our patients live as peaceful and as fulfilled a life as possible.

Do read this book. It opened my eyes to many reasons for the increasingly stressful environments we live in now, and made me understand why the enormous inequalities we see in the world today inevitably lead to increased ill-health. We need to strive for greater equality for the sake of the health of all, not just of the poor.

This reminds me again of what my Indian friend, Lotika, asked me: 'Why do you in the West want to be happy? We just accept.' And this is what even the poorest Indians sleeping on the streets do, as I observed them as they smilingly made way for me on the pavements, and pointed out helpfully where I had to go as I stood waiting for a taxi at Delhi station. I learnt a lot from that. I could not imagine the same thing happening in this country now. It is more likely that, in the same situation, far from being offered help, my handbag would be snatched from me.

◇◇◇◇◇◇◇◇◇

# 30 MARCH 2014
## *We all want to be heard*

I am off to China again with Mei and Guy in a week. And as usual before I go, I like to think of what stage I have reached in my own approach to my practice, and what will be the main theme around which we will build the two weeks of our seminar over there. The title which came to my mind this morning was: '*We all want to be heard.*'

It sounds so simple, put in that way, but actually it is one of the most difficult things of all for us to feel secure enough in our relationship to our hearer to have the courage to open up sufficiently so that what we say reflects truly what we feel, and therefore what is heard by our hearers is truly what we would like them to hear. What is so important for a good five element practice is that a patient must feel they can reveal what they are really feeling whilst knowing that what they reveal is being heard and understood properly. All too often, even in the caring professions, patients' words become distorted by hearers' preconceptions.

So my two weeks with my Chinese students will centre on the importance of allowing a patient sufficient space and time to feel emotionally safe with us, and ensuring that for our part we do not cast our own shadows over our patients so that what we hear is a distortion of the reality. When a patient feels that what they are telling us is being heard as they want us to hear it, this allows the elements within them to express themselves freely. When we cloud a patient's elements through incomprehension, we will not perceive them as they truly are, and will therefore be unable to respond to their needs. Elements can so easily disguise themselves, and, like snails under attack, draw back into their shells when they feel misunderstood. And this inevitably distorts our diagnosis.

I will use these thoughts as the foundation for our two weeks in Nanning. This is all the more important because Chinese culture places no emphasis on the importance of allowing patients to open up emotionally, and Chinese practitioners have to be encouraged to dare to take their first tentative steps in this direction. I well remember an incident from a previous visit to China, when an acupuncturist asked me, 'But how do I learn to talk to my patients about their emotions?'

I hope that after a further seminar with us she will be given some more help on how to do this.

◇◇◇◇◇◇◇◇

## 6 APRIL 2014
### *A lovely Picasso saying*

I have just come across something which Pablo Picasso apparently said: 'One starts to get young at the age of 60.'

I love that. I am many years older than Picasso was when he said that, but I quite understand the feeling. And it sends me off to China today very young in heart, if slightly creaky in body.

◇◇◇◇◇◇◇◇

## 23 APRIL 2014
### *What I have learnt from my recent visit to China*

I always find it reassuring to receive confirmation of the universal nature of human qualities. This is something we usually take for granted in everyday life. Politicians, for example, assume that those they negotiate with experience the same feelings they do, and are as horrified by the same injustices acting themselves out in far-flung places in the world out there as other politicians are. We think, too, that ordinary human folk, reading of tragedies such as the recent loss of the airliner or the ferry disaster, will be able to understand the sufferings of the bereaved at one remove. Unthinkingly for the most part, we assume that what others round the globe experience as suffering or joy mirrors our own experiences of suffering or joy.

Since as a five element acupuncturist my working life revolves around attempts to understand just what makes my patients suffer or be joyful, I am made particularly aware of my assumption of the universality of human emotions when I go to China, from where I have just returned. I wrote in a previous blog on 30 March, '*We all want to be heard*', which was about what I was expecting to be the focus of our seminar over there. I can now truly say that not only did the Chinese acupuncturists show that they did indeed hear what their patients wanted them to hear, but their responses to their patients reflected an increasing understanding and ability to respond to their patients' emotional needs.

There were about 70 acupuncturists at the seminar, of whom half were new to five element acupuncture. It was heart-warming to see how well those who were now practising five element acupuncture had integrated into their practice what they had learnt before. The comforting impression I returned with was a mixture not only of deep satisfaction at how many acupuncturists are now treating only with five element acupuncture, but – and this is perhaps the most surprising aspect of it all – how much easier I always find it handing on my knowledge to Chinese acupuncturists than I used to do to my English students. As I told them in China, 'You are all already halfway there compared with European (and presumably also American) students, because an understanding of the elements is deeply embedded in all of you from the day you are born, while non-Chinese students have to learn what is initially an alien language from scratch.' I well remember an English student asking me at the end of her first year at SOFEA, 'But how do you know that there are things called elements?'

It is therefore a continuing delight to me to see how much of what I want to convey to others about the wonder of the elements' presence within all of us is understood by my Chinese listeners almost before I open my mouth to speak. I notice how relaxed this makes me feel, as though I am wandering in a landscape with familiar landmarks, rather than the often difficult terrain I have had to negotiate over the years as my five element beliefs encountered the surprisingly sceptical opinions of my TCM colleagues.

I am very fortunate indeed to be accompanied on my visits to China by two very dedicated fellow five element acupuncturists, Mei Long and Guy Caplan, Mei from the Netherlands and Guy from here in London. We have now been together over there twice as a group, and Mei and Guy have also taught there once more without me in November 2013 when I was recovering from my recent illness. We act as a very unified group, each of us having slightly different roles which complement each other. It helps that Mei is Chinese and can speak without requiring the help of a translator. I'm sure this is a welcome relief from the inevitably interrupted communications which Guy and I make as we wait for our words to be translated. Again, we were lucky to have two very good translators to help us, Caroline and Nuha, both themselves acupuncturists, and I noticed this time how many of the group understood more English than they admitted to, laughing at my jokes before they were translated. I think there is quite a lot of English study going on during our absences.

And there were many jokes. We had a very happy time indeed, working hard and playing hard, too – many lovely meals out, some karaoke evenings, and a festive atmosphere as though all of us were enjoying a holiday together. And this is how I think the Chinese group view their time with us – as one long drawn-out holiday experience. In a way, I do, too, returning refreshed and stimulated by the enthusiasm and warmth with which we are surrounded throughout our time there.

I am only just getting used to carrying my own bags, too. In China, I was not allowed to carry anything at all, a small group waiting patiently for us in the hotel foyer every day at whatever time we emerged from our rooms, ready to grab my bags and lovingly accompany us the 100 yards or so to the centre where we taught. I can't remember the last time anybody helped me carry my bags in England!

◇◇◇◇◇◇◇◇

# 5 MAY 2014
## *A patient's comments*

Over the years I have become used to patients telling me things after treatment such as, 'Now I feel more myself again' or 'I know now who I am.' Yesterday I had another heart-warming example of five element acupuncture's ability to reach to the very heart of our needs as human beings, when a five element acupuncturist colleague told me how moved he had been when a patient described the effect of treatment in these words: 'I feel as if I've come into myself.'

I think that is such a lovely way of saying what we would all want to feel: that we have 'come into ourselves'. And how moving that what five element acupuncture can do is help our patients achieve that. In so doing, it also helps its practitioners achieve much the same thing, but by a different route, that of the therapist. When I feel a treatment I have given has helped my patient, I feel more fully myself.

◇◇◇◇◇◇◇◇

# 25 MAY 2014
## *The Chinese learn to hug each other*

Today's newspaper yielded yet another interesting snippet. An article from *The New York Times International Weekly* had the intriguing title 'Chinese unwind with a hug and a song'. Apparently, the Chinese are 'finally learning to hug each other' – although, from my own experience in China, they already know how to hug with great enjoyment.

Or perhaps it is that I have just met those who have spent time looking at the elements, and have had their interest in emotional responses stimulated by being told to observe what each element offers. Most people, this article appears to indicate, 'have been slow to embrace the embrace'. Liu Lihong told the class I was teaching that 'we need more Fire here'. In the case of hugs, it is probably more Earth that is needed, since I think hugging is much more a response to one of the Earth element's needs, which is to draw people close to them.

The article said that 'Recently it seems like everyone is hugging. Friends are hugging. Family members are hugging… The tables are turning… Schools are now conducting classes in emotional intelligence. For homework, children have been assigned to hug their parents.'

This trend towards learning to be unafraid to show emotions may be part of the reason why my Chinese five element students are so keen to learn all about the emotional manifestations of the elements, and enjoy doing exercises which help train them in learning to detect emotions both in themselves and in their patients.

◇◇◇◇◇◇◇◇◇

# 27 MAY 2014
## *The spacing of treatments: An art in itself*

I have just spent a happy few days in Berlin with two very dedicated German five element acupuncturists, Christian and Thomas. This was very stimulating, both culturally, because I saw more of Berlin on this, my second, visit, and from an acupuncture point of view, as it always is.

It was during a day spent looking at patients together that I was made aware once more of the importance of the question of the spacing of treatments as representing an essential, but often overlooked, aspect of how we help our patients.

I don't think that we pay enough attention to this in the normal course of events. At the start of a patient's treatment, I expect we all tend to give them a number of weekly treatments, normally something like six or so, and then we tend to space treatments more widely from once every 2–3 weeks to monthly and eventually to once a season or longer. It is what happens as we move further on in treatment that problems can arise. I was made aware of this again by one of the questions I was asked. How was the practitioner to deal with a patient who, he said, 'insisted' on weekly treatments whilst also maintaining that treatment was not helping him in any way?

We have various ways of assessing the effect of treatment. There are our own observations as to whether we notice any changes or not, and then there are the patient's own assessments of how treatment is going. Usually, these two sets of observations will coincide. Problems only start when the two differ, as, for example, if the practitioner notices how much better the patient looks, or the changes he/she is making to his/her life, and yet the patient him/herself says that there has been no change at all. We cannot try to persuade the patient by saying things like 'But you seem to be walking better' or 'You have not been talking about your family problems as much', because that is denying the patient the right to make their own assessment of what they consider constitutes improvement. On the other hand, we may be concerned that the patient is choosing not to acknowledge that there have been changes for other reasons. These may include such things as a fear that we are 'giving up' on them, or, more subtly, as part of some kind of a hidden power struggle between the patient and us. Some people can be unconsciously reluctant to accept the help of others.

How do we as acupuncturists get over this difficulty? If the relationship between our patient and us has been well grounded from the start, there should be no problem, as the patient's strengthened energies give them sufficient support gradually to do without our help. But if something in this relationship has tilted it towards over-dependence on us or otherwise distorted it, it may become more difficult gradually to hand control back to the patient. We may, for example, allow our patients to contact us too often between treatments by phone or now increasingly by email, something I was guilty of in the early days of my practice, because I felt I always had to be there to help my patients whenever they needed me. This can make it all too easy to blur the necessary lines of separation between patient and practitioner that make a healthy relationship possible.

We must never forget that our aim must always be to reach a point where we step back and treatment is no longer needed, the point where patients are now able to maintain balance by themselves. If we are having difficulties with working out how gradually to space out treatments for patients we can see require less treatment, we should examine our relationship with them to see if we have encouraged an over-reliance on us, and, if so, start gently to take steps to encourage the patient to greater independence. Of course, as with everything relating to our patients, our approach to each one will be different, and must be adapted to their individual needs. With one patient, treatments may remain weekly for much longer than with another. At each stage we have to assess whether our relationship to our patient is adapting flexibly to that patient's needs, and not depend upon a fixed formula for the spacing of appointments.

◇◇◇◇◇◇◇◇

## 29 MAY 2014
### *Returning the spirit to acupuncture in China*

*(Article submitted to* The Acupuncturist, *the newsletter of the British Acupuncture Council, as an introduction to the lecture I will be giving at the BAcC Annual Conference in September 2014)*

We are used to thinking of the transmission of traditional Chinese medicine as being a form of one-way traffic passing from East to West, but somewhat to my initial surprise, I have become a key factor in its journey in the opposite direction, from West to East. Specifically, it has become my task to take the first steps in helping five element acupuncture build a bridge back to its land of birth, China.

Over the years, China has made many different, often contradictory attempts to try to integrate its traditional form of medicine within the framework of Western medicine or to find ways of making Western medicine fit within it. It has never been quite clear whether it should view it as a powerful indigenous medical system on a par with, or even superior to,

Western medicine, or as a more primitive branch of medicine which Western medicine had in many ways superseded. This uncertainty has hovered over China's at times almost schizophrenic approach to its traditional medicine, and is one of the reasons for the confusion which this still causes, not only in China but to practitioners of Chinese medicine round the world. In other words, can Chinese traditional medicine be viewed as a stand-alone, intellectually coherent form of medicine based on more than 2000 years of continuous practice, or has the appearance of Western medicine in the past 100 years or so demoted it to an inferior, ancillary role?

It will be obvious from my writings and my teachings that I am utterly convinced of the former, but sadly I am not sure how far my view is shared by many of its practitioners either in China or the rest of the world.

Through a series of what could seem to have been coincidences, but which I regard now as clearly defined steps along a path that has guided me throughout my long association with acupuncture, I was led to meet Professor Liu Lihong at the Rothenburg conference in Germany a few years ago, together with his very good friend and translator, Heiner Fruehauf. Liu Lihong is described as being the most important Chinese medicine scholar of the younger generation in present-day China. His book *Sikao zhongyi* (*Contemplating Chinese Medicine*) became a bestseller when it was first published in 2003. It represents the first treatise written in China that openly discusses the shortcomings of TCM education in China.

I was then invited by him to give a seminar on five element acupuncture to acupuncturists at his research institute in Nanning in South China in November 2011, the first of five seminars I have given there to a growing number of acupuncturists. At my last visit in April, Professor Liu, who is himself a scholar of the classics, when introducing me to the class of 70 acupuncturists, said:

The seed of five element acupuncture is a very pure seed. I think it originates directly from our original classic Lingshu, 'Rooted in Spirit' (Chapter 8 of Lingshu), or 'Discourse on the law of needling' (Chapter 72 of Suwen). That is to say it fits easily within the Neijing. It is therefore not created from nothing. It has its origin in the far-distant past and has a long history. The seed which underlies its practice is very pure. For many good reasons, this seed has now returned to its homeland and started to germinate. In Nora's words, its roots have started to penetrate downwards.

I have been invited to give a keynote lecture on *'Returning the spirit to acupuncture in China'* at the British Acupuncture Council (BAcC) conference on 26 September 2014, when I will be describing in greater detail the process by which the roots of five element acupuncture are being encouraged to grow steadily stronger in China.

◇◇◇◇◇◇◇◇

# 22 JUNE 2014
*A testimony to how much the practice of five element acupuncture is helping one of my Chinese students*

The following is taken from an email from Caroline in Chengdu, who translates my blog for her fellow practitioners:

From the day on which I was helped by FEA [five element acupuncture], I've decided to learn FEA well and help more people. Because I have experienced the magic of FEA myself, which successfully helped me solve my family problem, I never had any problem of believing in FEA. I believe that the principle on which it is based is truth. And if I cannot cure people, the problem lies in me, not the principles of FEA. So I gave up learning to become a better herbalist, I just focused on FEA. It was not an easy change to make, but I struggled on. After one year of practising, I can now feel that I'm much more relaxed, hence I can pay more attention to my patient, and think less about the element. I learned how to have a better relationship with my patient, and learned a lot from them about how to become a better acupuncturist and a better person. And the more patients I see, the more information I can put in my library (of examples of elements), that's how I find myself getting a deeper understanding of the elements compared to one year ago. There is still a long long way to go, but I'm not in a hurry, it's a lifetime of learning, and I know that my patients will help me, thanks to all of them!

And translating your blogs helped me a lot too! Other people may just glance over it or read it once, while I will think every sentence over and over just to get a deeper understanding and find a better way to translate it. So after translating your blog, I can almost recite it! The whole process is like chewing your teachings and digesting it and making it mine. People may think my translating helped them, but honestly I think I'm the one who gain most.

I'll keep learning because it is such a happy and rewarding thing!

◇◇◇◇◇◇◇◇

# 25 JUNE 2014
## *Enjoying the ridiculous (yet again)*

Here's an amusing advertisement which I saw on my walk through London. Apparently, you can buy 'Invisible Personal Clothing'. My mind boggled at the thought of all those people walking around naked in invisible clothes, like the Emperor in his New Clothes. And apparently paying enough for the privilege of doing this to pay for a shop and its shop-front!

◇◇◇◇◇◇◇◇

# 2 JULY 2014
## *A lovely quote by Nietzsche*

I love finding these little snippets of other people's thoughts which illuminate my life. Here's one from the German philosopher Nietzsche, which I found in, of all things, a detective story:

> It's better to regret what you have done than what you never did.

This is a profoundly Metal thought. The life of those of the Metal element revolves around their deep need to assign to things their true value, and has as its necessary accompaniment the regret they may feel if they do not assess things correctly.

◇◇◇◇◇◇◇◇◇

# 2 JULY 2014
## *Never assume that we know how others feel*

We make all sorts of assumptions about other people, since we usually see them from our own perspective. It requires great insight and humility to try to step out from under the shadows each of us cast around ourselves and try to move into the sphere of another person. Unfortunately, we often delude ourselves that we understand another's viewpoint, whereas we are simply using our own viewpoint from which to judge theirs.

We must learn never to assume that we know anything about anybody else until we have proof from them that they are as we think they are. This is the secret of being a good therapist, and also, of course, of being a good parent, partner or friend.

◇◇◇◇◇◇◇◇◇

# 12 JULY 2014
## *Giving advice to patients*

I have just received an email from a Chinese acupuncturist asking how she can improve the skills needed to help her patients cope with their problems. She writes:

> How to interact with our patients is very subtle and skilful, and a very challenging task for us practitioners. I really wish I could do better on this, but I don't know how I could improve… [Their] problems are so

tricky that I always have no suggestion to give. I even sometimes don't know how to comfort them when they are sad. I wish I could say something to make them feel better!

I am sure that every practitioner can relate to what she says, for these are issues we have all struggled with in our practices, and no doubt continue to struggle with. There is no one approach that will suit all practitioners, because we will each have worked out our own way of dealing with our patients. As with everything we do, our own guardian element will shape our interactions with our patients and determine the nature of these interactions. Some practitioners will be much more hands-on in their approach than others (perhaps those with Fire as their element), whilst others will be much less so, giving their patients more room to breathe as it were (perhaps those with Metal as their element). No particular approach is better than any other, provided that the practitioner is aware at all times of how far what they are doing and saying matches their patient's needs.

Of course, this is where experience comes to our aid. If I think back on the years of my practice, I realize that there were many occasions when my own very hands-on approach disturbed some of my patients, where allowing a little more space between us would have given them the time they needed to work out their own solutions to their problems. As with any profession, we can only learn by hit and miss, and only experience will teach us how much advice it is helpful to give our patients, and what kind of advice this should be. As I mentioned in my previous blog of 2 July (*Never assume that we know how others feel*), we have to be careful not to assume anything about our patients.

Finally, it is helpful to remember that we are not there to solve our patients' problems; only they can do that. Our help must focus on offering treatments which bring greater balance to their elements, and then allow these to do the work.

◇◇◇◇◇◇◇◇◇

# 22 JULY 2014
## *Treating the whole person*

I've just read a very interesting article in *The Observer* with the title 'Over-treatment is the greatest threat to western health'. It ends with a quote from the 'visionary American physician and social activist Hunter Adams', who said, 'When you treat a disease, sometimes you win and sometimes you lose. But I guarantee you, when you treat a person, whatever the outcome, you always win.' The article finishes with the words, 'It's time for real "whole person" care.'

This is a subject very dear to my heart, as somebody who regards 'whole person' care as the main factor in helping our patients regain their health and balance. Having myself recently emerged successfully from a life-threatening condition (a subdural haematoma of the brain), with all that it has entailed of Western medical care, by far the most important aspect of the care I received was its 'whole person' aspect, the love of family and friends, and the caring attention of the medical staff.

But I remember thinking to myself when I returned back to normal life that what I had most wanted to be asked by the numerous medical personnel who surrounded me was the simple question 'How are you coping with this?' I was constantly asked about my physical well-being, but not about how my spirit was responding to the situation I found myself in. And, for me, this was what was troubling me most.

The best example I have ever encountered of the kind of question I would have responded eagerly to was that of a very junior nurse at some hospital visit a few years ago who said at the end of a diagnostic procedure I had undergone, 'You hate this, don't you?' And I certainly did. She had paid me the kind of close attention we should all pay our patients, and had made what in five element terms would have been considered to be an excellent diagnosis, saying just the right thing I wanted to hear. My immediate response was relief that here was somebody who saw *me* and understood my needs. This remains for me an illustration of what each of our patients would like from us. Each must hope their practitioner will have sufficient insight to see their unique needs and have the ability to respond appropriately to these needs, as this young nurse did to mine.

◇◇◇◇◇◇◇◇◇

# 11 AUGUST 2014
## *Writing and reading as acts of creation*

I am delighted once again to have chanced upon another good book, *We Are All Completely Beside Ourselves* by Karen Joy Fowler, which has made me see life from a different perspective, as should all good books. The only tiresome thing about it is its long-winded title, one of the many similar titles with which new books are often for some reason now burdened, perhaps to make them stand out from the crowd, but which, because of their long-windedness, slip from my memory immediately.

Apart from being beautifully written, it is also beautifully constructed with a startling shift of perspective midway through which sent me straight back to the beginning again to see whether I had missed some pointers that should have alerted me to this surprising development.

I learn about life as I read, and I also learn about life as I write. My writings, as, for example, of this blog, do not merely repeat thoughts I already have, but form stages in the process of developing these thoughts, which would not therefore see the light of day without the act of writing them down. It feels as though I am drawing these thoughts from within me as I write. Each then becomes a tiny act of creation, so that often as I read afterwards what I have written I surprise myself, as though I am reading something new written by somebody else.

◇◇◇◇◇◇◇◇

# 14 AUGUST 2014
## *I am a technophobe*

I am frightened of modern technology and the speed with which it changes. In the old days, hardly had I got used to the old VHS tapes when I had to learn how to use CDs, and now there are DVDs and smartphones and tablets and all manner of ways of listening to the radio and TV or downloading programmes I have missed. To me, it's a bewildering array of complex bits of equipment, all of which need to be plugged in somewhere to be charged or to be connected in strange ways I don't understand. And all of which, I am told by younger people as they manoeuvre their way seamlessly through it, are apparently there to make my life easier. This is not to mention social networking, such as Facebook and Twitter, which adds yet a further dimension to what I could do.

In the past, I have always called upon family and good friends to help me navigate my way through what I see as very choppy waters, but surely it is high time for me to confront my fears and at long last learn how to use my iPad, which I've had now for more than a year, rather than looking at it apprehensively each morning as I dutifully charge it up before putting it aside unused for another day.

So today I have finally decided to contact somebody who calls himself a computer geek and provides a one-man support system for people like me. Dare I lift the phone to ask for help, or will I leave it for another day, as I have left it for so many days?

As they say: 'Watch this space!'

◇◇◇◇◇◇◇◇

# 19 AUGUST 2014
## *We are becoming obsessed with ourselves*

I am trying to understand why people seem to feel such an increasing need to take photos of themselves, 'selfies', wherever they are, particularly with famous people. And I am also aware of how often people walking along the street turn towards shop windows to look at themselves. And not only look at themselves briefly to see whether they are looking alright, but repeatedly looking into window after window as they walk along the street. Sitting in the bus recently, I amused myself by watching how often those passing by on the street or standing at the bus stop looked at themselves in the bus window behind which I was sitting.

It seems as though the world has become a mirror in which everybody searches for their own reflection. Is this self-obsession with their own images a way of convincing themselves that they exist? And constantly taking photos of ourselves and looking at ourselves whenever we glimpse a reflection of ourselves is certainly a form of obsession. It can't be healthy to spend so long in observing oneself, rather than interacting with the world around us in a more fruitful, less selfish way. We are beginning to lose our awareness of others in looking so much at ourselves, as though we are living in isolation from one another.

I think back some years and realize that streets were usually lined with buildings which had smaller windows placed higher up the walls. You would be lucky if you could see yourself at all, and certainly not the whole of yourself. This craze for observing ourselves is therefore made much easier by the huge plate-glass windows all modern buildings now have, which show us from the crown of our head to the tips of our toes.

So mobile phones which overwhelm us with their noise and their insistent demands to be answered immediately wherever we are, as though the messages they send out are more important than any communication with those we are actually talking to, have blighted us in yet another way, by providing the cameras through which we can observe ourselves uninterruptedly all day long for as long as we want to. It seems we are beginning to prefer images of ourselves to our real selves.

◇◇◇◇◇◇◇◇◇

# 20 AUGUST 2014
## *How much reality can we stand?*

I have always loved the quote from TS Eliot's *The Four Quartets*: 'Humankind cannot bear very much reality.' And I am particularly aware of the truth of this as I prepare to plunge into today's newspaper, dreading yet another dose of all-too painful reality as I read what is going on in one country on the earth after another, and my heart bleeds for the people fleeing destruction with nowhere to go.

There seems to be nothing but misery in the world wherever I look, except when, with relief, I happen upon a TV programme showing some sport. Recently, it has been the Commonwealth Games and a cricket Test match which, to my and everybody's surprise, England won.

I think watching sport on TV keeps me sane, a form of extreme escapism which lightens the weight of the world upon my shoulders. And soon, an eagerly awaited event, golf's Ryder Cup. It happens to coincide with my talk at the British Acupuncture Council conference at the end of September, but having now learnt how to watch TV on my iPad, I will be able to catch glimpses of it at intervals between some more serious acupuncture input.

Perhaps already I am slightly less of a technophobe than I was when I wrote my blog on 14 August.

◇◇◇◇◇◇◇◇

# 1 SEPTEMBER 2014
## *The effect of treating a Window on an Inner Fire person*

I always love getting feedback about the effect of treatment from patients, and never more so if this is immediately after needling.

I treated a long-standing patient with Inner Fire as their guardian element (the Small Intestine, rather than the Heart). He always loves having his Windows needled, either II (SI) 16 or II (SI) 17, and occasionally both together when he feels the need for an acute sense of vision. Today I needled II (SI) 16.

He told me that immediately I had treated this point, his sight cleared. His vision had felt a bit blurred before, but it was now as if a veil had been lifted.

How lovely when we get confirmation of what an official can offer, and especially what a specific point adds to that official's effect. No element is more self-aware than the inner aspect of Fire. As we know, it is the supreme sorter, and as we needle it, it immediately starts sorting out what its reaction to treatment is.

◇◇◇◇◇◇◇◇◇

# 5 SEPTEMBER 2014
## *An example of the insensitivity of modern medicine*

I am often appalled by the insensitivity the medical profession can show towards its patients. Hidden within the well-intentioned aim of ensuring that patients are not banished from any discussion about what the future course of an illness is thought likely to be, doctors have started to err on the side of telling patients too much about the possible implications of some slight symptom or some tiny deviation from the normal in the results of some medical test or other. In so doing, they seem to forget that they are handing over the kind of information which is likely to frighten their patients.

I recently heard an example of this. A friend of mine went for a general check-up to a newly appointed doctor at her medical practice who conscientiously read through all her notes to familiarize himself with what was wrong with her. She had had a slight stroke some years back and was on medication to stabilize her heart. The doctor looked up from his notes, and said, 'You realize, don't you, that it says here that you are likely to get Alzheimer's at some point in the future.' Apparently some research had shown a correlation between having a stroke and Alzheimer's.

I asked my friend how hearing this had affected her. She is a very balanced, practical person with a good deal of understanding of medical matters and a sensible approach to her own health, certainly not the sort of person who would indulge in worrying excessively about what the future held for her. But she said that, despite her best efforts to ignore what she had been told, his words were still preying on her mind and had changed her approach to how she viewed her health. And yet there was no indication whatsoever of her having the slightest symptom of Alzheimer's, nor was there any medical or lifestyle advice which the doctor could have suggested to reduce the 'likelihood' of it occurring in the future. So what possible purpose, apart from making her fearful, had telling her this served?

My father, who was a doctor, always said that he had seen so many miracles in his long medical practice that he learned never to predict the course of an illness, and to take away hope was in effect condemning a patient to an earlier death. A little bit of hope was taken away from my friend yesterday by those few words spoken no doubt with the best of intentions, but unfortunately with the worst of results.

We should never take away a patient's hope. We don't have to pretend, even if it is obvious that a person is close to death, and we need to answer truthfully if asked, but if a patient wants to pretend that they have more time than we think they have, that is their right. And if hope allows them to feel a little better, however ill they are, they are likely to live a little longer, and perhaps die more peacefully.

◇◇◇◇◇◇◇◇

# 14 SEPTEMBER 2014
## *The Seven Ages of Man (and Woman)*

I have always liked to see the five elements as each embodying one of what are known as the Seven Ages of Man (though two of those ages are shared between the five elements). If we think of human life as circling in stages from birth to death, each life forms a similar progression to that of the elements, as it passes from its beginnings in Water on to Wood, to Fire, to Earth, to Metal and finally back to Water again. As Shakespeare puts it in Jacques' famous soliloquy in *As You Like It*:

> All the world's a stage,
> And all the men and women merely players:
> They have their exits and their entrances;
> And one man in his time plays many parts,
> His acts being seven ages. At first the infant…

And finishing with:

> … Last scene of all,
> That ends this strange eventful history,
> Is second childishness and mere oblivion,
> Sans teeth, sans eyes, sans taste, sans everything.

I see each phase of this circle of life as imparting its own quality to that life, each adding the quality of the element which it represents to those whose guardian element it is. There will therefore always be something of the child in a person with Wood as their guardian element, as there will be something of the exuberant joyfulness of the young adult emerging into the wider world of the adult in all Fire people, whatever their age. Each Earth person will show something of the mature adult throughout their life, as will a young Metal person show something of the wisdom of those approaching old age even in childhood. Water, always the most mysterious of all elements, the beginning and end of all things, will show both the naivety of the child which Wood always shows and the age-old wisdom of those living at the end of their days, which Metal hints at.

If a five element practitioner is unsure which element dominates in one of their patients, and they are unable to get enough information from their five senses to point towards one element, an attempt to see their patients in terms of how they appear in relation to the kind of stage of life they represent is a further way of helping our diagnosis. In my book *Keepers of the Soul,* I gave the example of my mother, definitely of the Wood element, as showing a childlike enjoyment of life at nearly 90 years of age, and I have a Metal son who I turn to to put me right about decisions in my life which my Fire element does not appear mature enough to make.

In this context, it is interesting to note the emotional ages of the friends we choose. I have always chosen those who are further along the cycle of the elements than me, predominantly the Metal element. I notice, too, that other people's choices of friends reflect something about the need for their own element to receive sustenance often from an element not their own which stimulates them.

I have never made a statistical survey of people's elements compared with the elements of their friends; this would indeed prove an almost impossible task, given that we need to treat a person for some time before really being sure of their element. But I suspect that many of us choose friends from amongst elements other than our own. I have always certainly done so, because, I have decided, I do not wish to have to observe in my friends the weaknesses I see in myself.

# 1 OCTOBER 2014
## *Element-watching with the Ryder Cup*

As everybody knows who has read this blog, I enjoy watching sport as a pleasant diversion from the horrors of much of what is going on out there in the world at the moment, and also because sportspeople reveal their elements much more clearly when under the extreme stresses competitive sport subjects them to.

So I have been watching the Ryder Cup, mostly on playback, since I was up at the British Acupuncture Council's annual conference for part of the weekend. And much of my watching has concentrated upon the Fire element, because not only is the leading golfer of the day, Rory McIlroy, most obviously Fire, but so is another well-known golfer, Sergio Garcia. So watching them together was a supreme example of the qualities particular to the Fire element. Not only did they stoke each other's Fire up so that they seemed to be having a little party between them all the time they played, but their joy also lit up the crowds watching them.

If you are unsure about what exactly distinguishes the Fire element from other elements, you can do no better than playing back those parts of the Ryder Cup from the TV programmes showing them in action. Watching these two golfers will teach you more about how to recognize the Fire element than any number of words. They are examples of how Fire lights up both itself and those around them, and I can guarantee that you will not be able to stop yourself smiling when you watch them. Only the Fire element will have this effect.

And then compare the effect these two people have on the crowds and on you with other golfers not of the Fire element

– for example, the American golfer Phil Mickelson. I think his element is Water, and though he is very warm towards the crowds and encourages their participation, he does not make me feel that I want to smile in the same way as I do whenever Rory McIlroy pops up on the screen. And there was also a rather angry Wood golfer I had never seen before, called Patrick Reed, who is also worth watching as providing a useful comparison with Rory McIlroy's and Sergio Garcia's Fire and Mickelson's Water.

Of course, since I don't treat any of these people, I always have to remind myself and those reading this blog that I cannot be sure that I am diagnosing the right elements. I therefore offer my diagnoses with the usual humility. But it's important that those of us who have been looking at the elements for many years (30, in my case) offer their expertise to those who are just starting on the road of five element acupuncture. I am more likely to be right now than I was 30 years ago when I started on this journey.

◇◇◇◇◇◇◇◇

# 27 OCTOBER 2014
## *Always query your diagnosis*

I woke this morning with a warm feeling in my heart. Yesterday we had another one of our very successful and satisfying seminar days which I share with Guy Caplan.

I always like to focus these days on diagnosing the elements in patients our participants want help with, or, as this time, diagnosing the participants themselves who want a clearer picture of their own element. You will note that I say 'a clearer picture' rather than a definite diagnosis.

This is something I insist upon, because I am so aware that a diagnosis can initially only be a tentative hypothesis and awaits confirmation from the way in which a patient responds to treatment. In other words, we are never sure that we have the right guardian element until that element has shown us, through its positive reaction to treatment, that this treatment is directed in the right place along the circle of the elements.

I know that hovering over all five element acupuncturists is the picture of JR Worsley interacting with a patient for a few minutes, and then turning to us with an immediate diagnosis of one element. This picture can delude us into thinking that every diagnosis we make should be equally fast. But, as JR told us as students, it had taken him more than 40 years' hard work to get to the stage he had reached. We would all be able to do the same, he said, once we had the same number of years' practice behind us. So those of us with far fewer years' experience will have to accept that tracking an element down to its source in a patient takes more than just a few minutes, and very often many more than just a few treatments.

What I tell students is that no patient minds how long this takes, provided they feel our compassion for them. A practitioner, Jo, who has attended many of our seminars, has just sent me the following lovely quote: 'People don't care what you know, they want to know that you care.' As long as we show we care, a patient will trust us to know what we are doing and allow us the time to work out gradually which element we should address with our treatment. We must never allow ourselves to be hurried by our patients into feeling that things should be moving more quickly than they are. One of the things we were told as students was that it takes about a month of treatment for every year of illness. That does not mean continuous weekly treatments, but it is a helpful rule of thumb, and allows us to tailor our expectations to a more realistic level.

Once my patients have started treatment, I have noticed that very few of them, if any, seem to spend much time talking about their symptoms, but instead want to talk about their life in general. In fact, they often forget altogether why they originally came to see me, evidence that patients do indeed want 'care', and not necessarily a 'cure', although with care often comes cure, since usually the two are closely related.

Our next seminar will be in the spring. In the meantime, Guy and I are off to China again in mid-November. Our usual enthusiastic group of practitioners over there are again organizing a preparatory five element course for the people who will be attending for the first time so that we will be preaching already to the converted. And luckily the new edition of the Mandarin version of my *Handbook of Five Element Practice*, with its *Teach Yourself* supplement, is flying off the shelves over there, and will give Chinese practitioners new to five element acupuncture a firm foundation on which to base their practice.

◇◇◇◇◇◇◇◇

# 13 NOVEMBER 2014
## *Publication of my blog book:* On Being a Five Element Acupuncturist

I have just completed revising the final proofs of my latest book, *On Being a Five Element Acupuncturist*, which will soon be hot off the Singing Dragon press. I call it my blog book because it includes the majority of the blogs I have been writing since 2010, and represents four years' hard, but enjoyable work. I find that seeing the blogs in book form is very different from reading them online. Somehow by putting them together into a book brings something out from them as a complete text which differs from what I call the snippets which individual blogs represent.

Anyway, I, as a lover of books, and not a person who enjoys reading by Kindle, however necessary this can sometimes be – as, for example, when travelling to China – am enjoying seeing the blogs now in the permanent form of a book rather than the ephemeral form of a computer-driven blog.

The book can be ordered from Singing Dragon (*www. singingdragon.com*) for delivery in early January.

◇◇◇◇◇◇◇◇◇

# 13 NOVEMBER 2014
## *Sixth seminar in China*

Guy and I are off to China again on Sunday for my sixth visit there and Guy's fourth. I had to tot up on my fingers the number of visits, and was surprised to find they were as many as that. Luckily, there is now a non-stop British Airways flight from Heathrow to Chengdu where, again, we will be met by our lovely Chengdu group of practitioners. They shepherd us beautifully around from one airport terminal to another, and invite us out to a lunch in-between. Then on to Nanning, where Liu Lihong and his group of practitioners will be waiting for us at the airport, with the usual huge clusters of flowers and warm cries of greeting, rather to the bewilderment of the Chinese travellers surrounding us.

We have a leisurely first day to recover from our jet lag (13-hour flight!), and then the hard work begins. Each day is full to the brim with teaching, supervising treatments and trying to give all those coming for the first time some idea of their element. This entails observing them carefully throughout our two weeks there to see whether our initial diagnosis still feels alright, and, if not, trying to work out in double-quick time which other element it might be. This is not something for the faint-hearted, and, as I have said before, it takes some courage even to attempt a diagnosis under such very rushed and quite stressful conditions. I'm pleased, though, that at previous seminars I had sufficient time to correct any diagnosis I was not happy with. And if these same practitioners come again this time, Guy and I will double-check whether we are happy with our original diagnoses.

As usual, there will be more than 60 practitioners at the seminar, of which 40 have already been to previous seminars and 20 will be new people. I like the mix of the more experienced and the total novices, and love seeing how the more experienced are now gradually stepping more confidently into the role of teacher.

◇◇◇◇◇◇◇◇

# 1 DECEMBER 2014
## *Back from my sixth visit to China*

Each time I come back from China, I become increasingly aware of the importance tradition plays in its life and how much less this seems to be true of England. This was particularly so on this visit when I gave a talk to some 300 students of traditional Chinese medicine at the Guangxi University of Chinese Medicine. As I stood outside the lecture hall waiting to be introduced, I could hear the students in unison chanting a text appearing on the large screen behind the platform. I was told that this represented a passage from the writings of Sun Si Miao about the purity and sincerity of the great physician, which they recite each day before they start their classes. This is much as if medical students over here were daily to recite the Hippocratic Oath.

As they finished and I was led on to the platform, I felt that I was being ushered into the presence of a long line of Chinese practitioners stretching back many hundreds of years, much as I always feel that JR Worsley stands at my shoulder as I talk about five element acupuncture. This feeling was made even stronger by being asked to be photographed at the feet of a giant statue of Zhang Zhong Jing (150–215 AD), writer of the *Treatise on Exogenous Febrile Disease,* which towers over the campus. The sense of a long line of transmission of traditional medicine is undoubtedly and quite understandably much stronger in China, the country of its birth, than anything experienced in other countries. And it is now accompanied by a realization of the tragic discontinuity of these old traditions caused by the upheavals of its recent past.

This is why our visits are regarded by our hosts as a heartening reconnection to what has been lost. Five element acupuncture is seen as a pure form of traditional acupuncture whose roots lie buried deep in the Nei Jing and whose great trunk is now growing ever stronger new branches back in China.

I am so very delighted by increasing evidence of the rebirth of five element acupuncture amongst the many new students attracted to the seminars we have been giving over the past three years. It pleases me that the group of our first students are now themselves giving preparatory seminars to new students before we arrive so that we no longer need to teach the most basic principles of five element acupuncture, but can each time move on to a more advanced level.

There were 70 students in this latest group, half of them new and half practitioners who had come to previous seminars. Unfortunately, Mei Long could not be with us this time, so Guy Caplan and I had to work a little harder. I was asked how many more new students we could accommodate next time we go, which will be in April 2015, and I said as many as can fit into the new premises of the Tong You San He Centre where we teach. I understand this to be about 90–100. Since we include in each seminar somewhat hastily arranged diagnoses of each new student's guardian element, this represents a significant challenge to us. But it is a challenge which I have learnt we must accept, since to leave a new student of five element acupuncture with no idea at all of their own element undermines their confidence in what they are learning.

As groups of them line up for us to try to see what diagnostic pointers we can observe to help in our diagnoses, I always tell them that this is a very inadequate form of diagnosis, and not at all what they should be doing with their own patients, but that the time constraints we are working under make it the only possible one, given the numbers in our seminars. The students are therefore quite happy if later during the seminar, after watching them carefully, we decide to change our diagnosis. And each of them is given a treatment consisting of an Aggressive Energy drain and source points of the diagnosed element as a further way both of teaching them the basic simple tenets of our practice, and of allowing us to observe the effects of this treatment to help us assess whether we think our diagnosis is correct or not.

We came back, as usual, laden with presents, so that even though I took over a large batch of my books to give to any English-speaking practitioners in the group, and thought I would return with a half-empty suitcase, I was still overweight at the check-in desk!

# 1 DECEMBER 2014
## *Wood quote from* Anna Karenina

You could not have a better description of the qualities of the Wood element than that from this passage which I came across when reading Tolstoy's *Anna Karenina* in my hotel room in China.

> Spring is the time of plans and projects. And as he came out into the farmyard, Levin, like a tree in spring that knows not what form will be taken by the young shoots and twigs imprisoned in its swelling buds, hardly knew what undertakings he was going to begin upon now in the farm work that was so dear to him. But he felt that he was full of the most splendid plans and projects.

◇◇◇◇◇◇◇◇

# 11 DECEMBER 2014
## *The curse of the mobile phone*

I have written before about the way in which I think the use of mobile phones and other electronic equipment is having a negative effect upon human interactions. I am reluctant to condemn all these new inventions because in many ways they are miracles of human invention, but it is hard for me to see their good in a world now increasingly peopled by automaton-like figures peering into their screens with never an eye raised to acknowledge the presence of those they are passing by.

If you become used to allowing the demands of the mobile phone to control your life in this way, I wonder how this will affect human interactions in the long term. More and more people now appear to be compelled by their insistent ringing tones to give mobile phones priority over everything else, to the extent that they allow them to interrupt whatever social interactions are taking place at the time.

I was reminded of this at a restaurant I went to last week, where the owner said that she was quite happy for us to sit on as long as we wanted after we had finished our meal, because she was so pleased to find people who had not spent the whole of their meal shouting into mobile phones, as her other guests often do. She is appalled at the way these telephone conversations are conducted at high volume without consideration for other diners, but said, 'I can't tell people they mustn't use their phones because I would lose too many customers if I did.' Recently I heard the story of an irate diner, who, plagued by the incessant loud mobile conversation at the table next to his, had simply got up, grabbed the phone and thrown it into a large bowl of flowers where it bobbed about helplessly. 'You've spoilt my meal,' he said, 'so now I'm spoiling yours.' I certainly often have a strong inclination to follow suit, but I'm not sure I have this man's courage.

There appear to be very few people left who would still consider it rude to interrupt a conversation with a friend to answer their phones. And if we increasingly ignore those who are physically close to us as we respond to the demands of those disembodied voices on our machines, what effect will that have on human relationships in the future?

Why the need, too, for so much hurry? We have become slaves to these tiny machines.

◇◇◇◇◇◇◇◇

# 28 DECEMBER 2014
## *Happy end to 2014*

I like to end my blogs of 2014 on an optimistic note. And what could be happier in an age where people seem obsessed by ever more useless consumerism than to hear of the generosity of people towards those consigned to the bottom of the pile. And in London some of these are eking out a living selling the *Big Issue* on the streets. I have my own familiar group of *Big Issue* sellers for whom I keep a stash of coins ready in my pockets as I walk around London, but I found myself in an unfamiliar part of town walking past a seller I had not seen before. As he smiled at me, I asked him whether his takings for that day had been good. 'No,' he said, 'it seems that everybody is just hurrying past to do their Christmas shopping. But I must tell you about two lovely things that happened to me a few days ago. One of my regular customers came rushing up to me on his way to fly off abroad for Christmas, and pressed a £50 note into my hand. And not long afterwards, another person gave me £20. That was my lucky day, wasn't it?'

And I, too, was the surprised recipient of other people's kindness. In one of my favourite coffee houses, I decided to give myself a pre-Christmas treat of various goodies, and asked for the bill. The waitress said, 'I don't think you will be needing that,' and returned not with my bill but with a Christmas card from all the staff with my name on it. I don't know how they found out who I was, because I usually pay with cash, but I must have once paid with a credit card with my name on it. And they refused to let me pay for my little feast.

So there is more generosity around than there often appears to be on the surface. I left both the *Big Issue* seller and the café with a big smile on my face.

◇◇◇◇◇◇◇◇

# 28 DECEMBER 2014
## *2015 New Year's wish*

As 2014 draws to a close, signalling the end of another year of my life, I am made increasingly aware of the steady passing of time, like the annual tick-tock of the clock of my life, a form of countdown to its end. I don't find this a morbid thought – quite the reverse. It just sets me thinking about what I still have to do, and gives it an increasing urgency. This is becoming all the more pressing since my body is finally admitting to its increasing age, with the gradual diminution of all kinds of faculties I have so far taken for granted. Foremost among them is my hearing, which has always been a problem and is beginning now to affect my social life to the extent that I have to consider before joining others how far my struggle to hear what people are saying will affect my enjoyment of their company, and no doubt their enjoyment of mine, as I have to ask them to repeat what they have said. And then there are my creaking knees, about which the less said the better.

But, and here is the flipside to this, all these physical problems, which are after all minor compared with what many people are forced to suffer, persuade me that I have in a way to hurry up and do all that I feel I have to do before my body compels me to a full stop. Certainly, my mind appears to be more active than ever (at least nobody has so far dared tell me if this is not true!), though, as all of us notice as we grow older, our memory, particularly of names but certainly not of faces, begins to suffer. My sister, two years older than me, told me recently that she wanted to pack in as much travelling as she could 'whilst I still can', and I, too, want to do as much as I can whilst I still can. But the big question is not travelling, which I am continuing to do quite happily (off to China again in April for my seventh visit), but what to write!

The book of my blogs, to be called *On Being a Five Element Acupuncturist*, will appear in bookshops in January, and I want to organize a book launch for it, as a way of celebrating its completion but also as a good pretext for inviting many of those people from my days as Principal of the School of Five Element Acupuncture with whom I have lost contact in the years since I closed the school. I hope the reception room at our Harley Street clinic will be large enough to hold everybody. But after that, what?

I feel bereft without the project of another book to work on. Blogs such as the one I am writing now certainly help me formulate my thoughts, but I ask myself whether I have anything left to say about five element acupuncture, or is it more about life that I need to write? (And as I ask this question there flashes through my mind an odd thought about the way the Fire element walks, which was stimulated by watching Rory McIlroy, the golfer, in a re-run of some of the highlights of the Ryder Cup this year on TV, prompting me to write another blog about the elements.)

At midnight on New Year's Eve each year I make a pledge to try to complete a further aim which I set for myself for the coming year. I now only have about three days between now and the end of the year to discover what this year's wish will be. Will I manage to do it this year or not?

# 2015 BLOGS

# 2 JANUARY 2015
## *The need to write*

I love reading of people who, often to their own surprise, have found themselves spurred on to write, as though they have at some point in their lives found themselves unexpectedly before an open gate which beckons them out on to a landscape of words. I have just come across two heartening examples of this.

Katharine Norbury, who is just about to publish her first book, *The Fish Ladder: A Journey Upstream*, writes: '… suddenly I thought, "I've got something to say!", so I started saying it. At my age it's very relaxing to know there's something out there that has some of my philosophy and thoughts in it… I'm very happy that I've finally said something.'

And in the biography of a rather delightfully odd writer of detective stories, Suzette Hill, I found the following: 'At the age of sixty-four and on a whim, she took up a pen and began writing.'

I have written books about acupuncture and continue to write this blog which gives me the chance 'on a whim', as Suzette Hill says, to write about the odd thoughts I have. But I have never written anything in greater detail about my life, nor have I ever wanted to write anything fictional. As I said in my blog of 28 December 2014 (2015 New Year's Wish), apart from blog-writing, I seem to be facing a book made up of blank pages, as though they are waiting for me to write words upon them. But I am not yet clear what words these will be? I would like to be able soon to say that these blank pages are starting to fill up with my writing, and then be able to say with as much glee as Katharine Norbury does, 'I'm very happy that I've finally said something,' and, in my case, it would be truer to say 'something else'.

◇◇◇◇◇◇◇◇

# 7 JANUARY 2015
## *The qualities of a good physician*

Heiner Fruehauf has translated part of a very interesting passage from a 1000-year old text about the qualities of a good physician. To see the whole text, look at his website, www.ClassicalChineseMedicine.org.

> ... Every physician should be warm and dignified by nature, humble and respectful by disposition; polite in actions; soft and flexible in behaviour; devoid of self-aggrandizing attitude and without indulgence in pride and extravagance.

> ... Wealthy and poor patients should be treated with the same level of attention, and those with rank and those without social status should receive the same type of medicine.

> ... Nobody should ever be treated the same way – this principle was most important to the wise physicians of old.

These extracts are taken from his translation of *A Guide to Children's Health: Theoretical Discussions and Treatment Plans, 1156 AD.*

I have chosen a few passages which are particularly dear to my heart, the most important to me by far being the last, a precept, I notice, which is closest to the anonymous author's heart, too. 'Nobody should ever be treated the same way.'

This is one of the reasons why I love being a five element acupuncturist, and why some people find this too challenging a discipline. No five element acupuncturist can look up in a book to find a prescribed set of points for a set condition. Each person presents a unique challenge to the practitioner, a unique puzzle, a conundrum which needs to be solved anew at each treatment. The question each time must be 'What treatment should I give today which meets my patient's needs of today?' And I emphasize 'of today', because today's needs always differ from yesterday's, and differ even more widely from those I diagnosed when first I encountered my patient. Our anonymous author says, 'Nobody should ever be treated the same way,' and I would add, 'Nor the same way as they were treated when we last saw them.'

We may be delighted to see how the previous treatments have helped our patient, but we cannot then rest on our laurels and simply repeat what we have done so far. The patient coming to see us today is different from the one who came yesterday, or last week or last month. He or she has lived another cycle of minutes, days or weeks, and is thus a different person from the person to whom we bade farewell last time.

And I have often experienced a slight shock when the patient coming into my practice room today appears so different from the one who left me after the last treatment. Life has added another layer to them, and may either have further burdened them or lifted some of that burden, but will have altered, however slightly or radically, the interplay of the elements within them. Since time never stands still, the elements which reflect time's pressure upon us can in their turn never stand still. And thus our treatments, directed at these elements, have to adapt themselves to take account of these changes.

◇◇◇◇◇◇◇◇◇

# 15 JANUARY 2015
## *Rory McIlroy's walk*

Each fresh encounter with the elements, which occurs whenever I meet a new person, either fleetingly in the street or for longer in my practice room or in my social relationships, provides an opportunity to add to my knowledge.

An example of this occurred recently when I was casually watching some golf on TV (and everybody who knows me also knows not only how much I enjoy watching sport but, in particular, watching sportspeople often revealing surprising aspects of their true natures, and thus of their elements, under the stress of competition). I suddenly noticed the golfer Rory McIlroy's walk. I can best describe it as a kind of jaunty stride. It is certainly not a stroll, nor does it appear to be a form of hurrying, and yet I can find no better way of describing it than to say that he walks as though pushing the air aside in front of him, not in any way aggressively, but firmly. It is definitely a stride, but done with a kind of joyousness to it. Usually, he smiles as he walks. You feel that if you were in front of him, you would have to give way to allow this force of nature to pass by.

That set me thinking about the different ways the elements walk. McIlroy is so obviously an excellent example of the Fire element. He can't stop smiling and he can't stop making others laugh. When he and Sergio Garcia (another Fire person, although slightly more subdued Fire) were paired together in the 2014 Ryder Cup, it was like watching two young children larking around on the golf course, with a lot of touching and laughing and an atmosphere of sheer enjoyment almost at odds with the seriousness of the competition.

I then compared his walk with that of another competitor, Patrick Reed, whom I diagnosed as the Wood element. Wood, after all, is another very young, outgoing element, with perhaps an even more forceful signature than Fire as its hallmark. But Reed's walk, though firm, differed from McIlroy's because it did not have the same kind of joyous spring to it. It was more of a firm placing of one foot in front of the other, a kind of a stomp, like someone claiming that bit of ground for himself, so that he made me more aware of the force with which each foot landed on the ground. McIlroy's stride makes me aware of the top of his body, as his chest breasts the air in front of him, Reed's more of his feet conquering the ground. This may seem a little fanciful, but I don't think it is. Wood, after all, emphasizes the feet; Fire, the top half of the body.

This made me think about my own Fire stride. Did I have something akin to McIlroy's walk, and did other Fire people, too, or had my observation not revealed a characteristic peculiar to all Fire people but only to the one? I have not yet come to any satisfactory conclusion about this, but if anybody were to watch me walking along the street, they might be surprised to note how often I glance in shop windows as I try to catch myself in mid-stride to analyze how I am walking. Thus do I learn a little more about the elements each day.

◇◇◇◇◇◇◇◇

# 25 JANUARY 2015
*New words of wisdom*

I like to collect wise sayings, and today, to my delight, I have come across two, both of which have taught me something new.

Here they are: 'I'm getting angrier as I get older,' said by the artist Cornelia Parker, and a quotation from Tolstoy: 'We can know only that we know nothing. And that is the highest degree of human wisdom.'

The first, by Cornelia Parker, echoes something which I have only just become aware of, my own increasing sense of anger at the inequalities of this world. I only have to think of those rich people gathering in Davos now, all flying in with their private jets, and most of whom, I expect, live in gated communities to keep the starving hordes at bay, for this sense of anger within me to well over into a kind of fury that the poor and disadvantaged are expected to make sacrifices whilst the rich just add to their financial portfolios.

And, seen from the point of view of a five element acupuncturist, the Tolstoy quotation is an excellent reminder to me of something I always want to emphasize in my teaching. With every patient we see, we must always start from a position of absolute humility, of 'knowing nothing', because each is unique and teaches us something completely new.

I will leave my readers to decide whether either of these quotations resonate for them as they do for me.

◇◇◇◇◇◇◇◇

## 26 JANUARY 2015
### *Beckham's beard*

I find it fascinating to observe the influence certain famous people can have upon a whole generation. This is so in the case of David Beckham and his beard. I remember a time, now shrouded in the mists of quite a few years, when only a dedicated few wore beards, and certainly not footballers.

And then along comes David Beckham, a style icon if ever there was one, sporting one kind of beard after another, first just a discreet growth on the chin, followed by other kinds of adornments, and finally a thick bushy beard which certainly did him no favours. This has now been trimmed back to the kind of beard everybody is now wearing, in mimicry of him.

Once Beckham was seen with a beard, I noticed that they gradually started to sprout everywhere, until, now, particularly among footballers, it is almost odd to see a beardless face. And not just in this country, but throughout the world.

I wonder how far each bearded person thinks his type of beard suits him. To my eyes, some definitely do whilst others definitely do not. I think here of Gary Lineker on BBC TV, whose face appears to have shrunk behind his rather wispy beard, whilst others' beards suit them better.

I wonder, too, how far the women in these bearded men's lives like this new fashion. I know of one young man whose relationship has foundered on his girlfriend's insistence that he shave off his beard, and a wife who hated her husband's. They are, after all, really prickly!

And there is also the case of Beckham's tattoos, another fashion many footballers have followed!

I am now waiting for Beckham to shave off his beard to see whether the fashion will change again. I think the tattoos are here to stay.

◇◇◇◇◇◇◇◇

# 29 JANUARY 2015
## *A beautiful poem*

I am not a natural reader of poems. I have always found that I need to hear somebody reading them to me before I really understand their rhythm. But I have just been introduced by a poetry-writing friend to a poem by John Clare (1793–1864), one line of which has haunted me ever since. It is the third line of the poem, and I have decided that it will be good to exercise my brain by trying to learn the whole, quite short poem.

The line is from a poem called simply 'I am', and here are its first three lines, written down, to my delight, already from memory:

> I am, yet what I am none cares or knows;
> My friends forsake me like a memory lost:
> I am the self-consumer of my woes

(I got a few words wrong!)

I don't know why these lines swirl away in my mind as much as they do. I suppose that this is one of the secrets of good poetry. Its rhythms and its juxtapositions of oddly assorted words lead us away from the everyday into some distant realm of the spirit. 'I am the self-consumer of my woes' speaks to me in a way I don't really understand, but simply feel.

He was completely self-taught, working as a labourer in the fields to support his family, and then unhappily spent the last years of his life consigned to an asylum. I have just discovered that 'I am' was the last poem he wrote. He must indeed have felt that his friends had forsaken him 'like a memory lost', so that he had to become 'the self-consumer of his woes'.

Reading about his life, and its unhappy ending, I can at last begin to understand the meaning of these lines.

◇◇◇◇◇◇◇◇

# 22 FEBRUARY 2015
## *An important book*

I have just read an important book all should read, *The Internet Is Not the Answer* by Andrew Keen. As readers of my blog know, I am increasingly disturbed by the impact of what I call the electronic world upon us all. We are enveloped (literally) in it. Anything I do, where I do it, when I do it and what I do with it, can be tracked, as my life is monitored from minute to minute, my shopping preferences noted, my reading choices logged, my finances closely scrutinized and my telephone calls snooped on.

I am always surprised at the welcome given to all new inventions emerging almost daily from this electronic world, apparently with little thought given to any possible downside to them. The latest evidence for this is the attention the fashion world is now paying to designing clothes with inbuilt pockets for mobile phones and all the other computer equipment people now carry with them, and with a self-charging capacity so that as we walk along we can charge this equipment up without the need to find a socket somewhere to plug it in. We will in effect be charged into ourselves. I had to look at my diary to check whether I had skipped a few months and this was April Fool's Day!

Andrew Keen's book points to the many pitfalls of this electronic world, not only ahead of us, but, dismayingly, already all too evident here and now. The large all-powerful, all-devouring companies of Amazon, Google and the like already hold so much of our lives in thrall that it feels as though there is little any of us can do to counter their power except increasingly protest at this power and make, as I do, our own small gestures of protest. These include doing things like buying my books at a small local bookshop rather than through Amazon, and buying my newspaper from my small local newsagent rather than at Tesco's, so much more conveniently closer to hand.

So books like this one by Andrew Keen, based on very detailed, insider evidence of the terrifying consequences as all these huge monoliths gradually take over ever larger slices of our life, are essential reading, particularly for those, such as politicians, wielding more power than I can ever do. They do have the chance to halt the progression of these juggernauts over the land. But at least people are now increasingly awake to the injustice of their hiding away their huge profits in secret tax havens in such a way as to avoid paying taxes on them, and are demanding action on this. A small but, I hope, significant step.

◇◇◇◇◇◇◇◇

# 22 FEBRUARY 2015
## *The joy of being with other five element acupuncturists*

After depressing myself by writing the last blog, I am relieved to turn to a much happier subject for this blog, which is about another heart-warming seminar Guy Caplan and I gave yesterday at our clinic in Harley Street. I love the word 'heart-warming', a word close indeed to every Fire person's heart, such as mine, because it does feel as if my heart this morning is indeed warmer after a day spent in the presence of a group of dedicated five element practitioners and students.

We look at patients together, observe their treatments, include some practical work helping participants feel more confident about their clinical skills, and, most importantly of all, mull over together the problems we confront as practitioners. Mostly, though, we concentrate simply on making participants feel more confident in what they are doing, and helping them by making them aware that they are part of a family of five element acupuncturists. The main thing which I like to emphasize and which I hope they all take away with them are my two mantras: 'The simpler the better' and 'Points are messengers of the elements, not the message itself.'

I am constantly bewildered by the emphasis so many people now seem to put on points and point selection. When I trained all those years ago, we never seemed to worry about which points to select because the whole emphasis of training was on trying to find a patient's element. Once found, or at least once we had made our first decision about which element to address, we carried out the simplest of treatments: first, of course, AE drain, then source (yuan) points, tonification points, horary points, Associated Effect Points (AEPs – back shu points), interspersed, obviously, by clearing any blocks, such as Possession, Husband/Wife or Entry/Exit blocks. I don't remember us ever worrying about point selection, unlike present generations of practitioners who seem to spend an inordinate amount of time mulling over the actions of different points and when to use them, and disproportionately less time learning to look carefully at the elements of which these points are just the servants.

Another mantra of mine could be 'Find the element and the points look after themselves.' And if they don't yet look after themselves, because you are new to the world of five element acupuncture, then look at a copy of the new edition of my *Handbook of Five Element Practice*, published by Singing Dragon, which lists in careful detail the points on each element to be used at different stages of treatment.

So a day spent with my group of five element practitioners and students, all speaking the same language of the elements, is confirmation that at least in this corner of London the spirit of five element acupuncture in its purest form continues to flourish. This confirmation has been given an additional boost by an email from one of the participants which I received at the end of the day, telling me how grateful he and other members of the group were to see 'how you simplify 5E acupuncture in a way that we can all get a real grasp of the elements'. Thank you, Dom, for those kind words.

◇◇◇◇◇◇◇◇◇

# 23 FEBRUARY 2015
## *Being an unashamed Luddite**

The world gets more and more bizarre to me, and more and more in thrall to all the computerized gadgets being invented by the day to satisfy some never-satisfied appetite for the new. I live near an Apple store and have seen the queues building up outside its doors on the days some new gadget is put on sale. Presumably, each of these must incorporate some additional feature considered essential by its buyers, a symbol of conspicuous consumption if there ever was one.

I am at the opposite end of this spectrum of a desire for new computer gadgets, having been lent an iPhone a short

---

\*    A person opposed to new technology

while ago only to hand it back when I could never learn its uses, and retreated back to a mobile phone apparently so outdated as to be out of the dark ages – and only used by me for emergencies. And then only reluctantly because I need to put on my spectacles to see what I am doing, which means ferreting around in a bag, and then, because of my bad hearing, being unable to hear the person I am trying to contact because of all the traffic noise. Admittedly, I am not a neutral observer of the computer scene, particularly when I am sitting close to somebody in a coffee shop who is engaged in simultaneous computer-driven activities, as I was a few days ago.

For there I am enjoying my morning coffee with my book open in front of me when a young woman rushes into the café, plonks herself down opposite me (and the tables are quite narrow and intended for groups of people sitting closely with each other), talking all the while on her phone. With one hand she holds the phone against her ear, with the other she fusses around in her bag to get out her laptop. Talking all the while and passing the phone from ear to ear as she tries to open her computer, at the same time somehow she manages to interrupt herself for long enough to place her order with the waitress. The she starts tapping the keys on her computer rather frantically, whilst taking off her coat. By now I am watching fascinated by her ability to multitask – to talk and to type and to take off her coat, but then comes the *coup de théâtre*. Her coffee and a plate of toast arrives, and somehow, to my amazement, by dint of moving the phone into which she is still talking from hand to hand, or holding it by her shoulder against her ear, she manages to release one hand enough to pick up a knife and butter her toast, admittedly rather clumsily, but still sufficiently to be able to snatch at it, interspersed by gulps of coffee, all the while still talking on the phone and tapping on the computer.

By now I am so jittery myself from all these frantic movements opposite me that I decide I have had enough and leave. I saw her again a few days later, still frantically engaged in all the same activities. Not once has she even exchanged a glance with me or the waitress serving her. She is in a networking bubble all on her own.

I wonder what this is doing to her Earth element, as it tries to take in and process the information pouring in to her through phone and computer, as well as the food and drink which is there to nourish her. I can visualize this poor element desperately trying to carry out its work, but not sure what to do first. It certainly didn't help my own Earth element, which couldn't process what I was watching, and I had to leave.

◇◇◇◇◇◇◇◇◇

# 1 MARCH 2015
## *Are we living in an age of Metal?*

I would recommend all of you to read a book by Andrew Keen, called *The Internet Is Not the Answer* (Atlantic Books, 2015). It sounds important warnings about the world we live in, and the risks we are running of remaining, not the free agents in a free world we like to see ourselves as, but ever more like slaves entrapped in a world controlled by the large corporations, such as Apple, Amazon and Google, whose power over us grows by the day.

The author points to a worrying aspect of today's world – our current obsession with ourselves. The rise of the mobile phone and Instagram have disturbing consequences, one of the most frightening being what he calls our 'self-centric culture', in which 'if we have no thought to Tweet or photo to post, we basically cease to exist'. And, 'The truth about networks like Instagram, Twitter, or Facebook is that their easy-to-use, free tools delude us into thinking we are celebrities.'

I have often thought that the electronic equipment most of us feel to be absolutely indispensable to our modern lives, and which is intended to link us ever more closely to one another, ironically leads instead to our distancing ourselves more and more from each other. The cameras in our mobile phones are encouraging us to look at each other through a lens, rather than in the eye. The messages we send are beginning to stop us speaking to one another, voice to voice. We now text rather than talk.

The young woman sitting opposite me in the café (see my last blog of 23 February) made no contact with anybody during the time that I watched her, all her human interactions being through her electronic equipment. It felt as though she lived in a bubble all on her own. As Andrew Keen says, 'The truth…is that we are mostly just talking to ourselves on these supposedly "social" networks… [It is] an Internet in which the more social we become, the more we connect and communicate and collaborate, the lonelier we become.'

Finally, to add to these rather depressing thoughts, a little comment by the writer Robert Macfarlane, whose lovely books about walking in nature and in the wild all of us should also read. In an article of his in *The Guardian*, I read that the new edition of the *Oxford Junior Dictionary* now includes words like 'chatroom' and 'broadband', but not 'bluebell' or 'kingfisher'. I also read that they are now discussing whether children should continue to be taught handwriting in school, presumably because it is assumed that they will no longer be using pen and paper but tapping away on their keypads to communicate. All these different developments underline the seismic changes going on around us. No doubt many of these may herald exciting new departures which we should welcome. Others, though, represent losses. I am sad that children's vocabularies may no longer include bluebells or kingfishers.

Are we perhaps starting to live in an age of Metal, that element which mourns the loss of what is valuable, and in its imbalance may cut us off increasingly from each other and from the world around us?

◇◇◇◇◇◇◇◇

# 2 MARCH 2015
## *A few thoughts on astrology*

My family knew a very interesting old Viennese man called Dr Oskar Adler, who has influenced me in some surprisingly different ways. He was what we call a polymath, one of those now rare breeds of multi-disciplined people with interests and training in widely ranging areas of life. He was a musician, a marvellous violinist who, I was told, had taught the composer Arnold Schoenberg the violin, a mathematician and – and this was where he most influenced me – a widely respected astrologer. I have on my bookshelves a copy of his large four-volume treatise on astrology (in German). It is beautifully written and very profound, one of those works which has given me deep insights into human behaviour.

I have a rather confused understanding of astrology. I think I would have described myself in the past as a sceptic, and yet time has changed me. One of the changes came about by attending a short astrology course in London years ago, when for the first time I began to appreciate that there were indeed individual human characteristics which could be symbolized by a person's relationship to the planets in the heavens. At first I needed a lot of convincing that this could be so, until the class was one day given the astrological chart of a famous anonymous person and was asked to try to work out who that person might be. To my utter surprise we came up with the correct answer (it was Princess Diana, much in the news at that time). We then compared her chart with that of Prince Charles. This comparison clearly showed that they were set on a collision course, aspects of the one chart clearly clashing violently with those of the other. This was my first venture into the arcane world of astrology. As a surprise by-product, it has added much to the understanding of human nature which my five element studies were teaching me.

There are 12 astrological signs and 12 officials spread between the five elements, though unfortunately we cannot equate one with the other. If we could, we would have an easy way of diagnosing an element simply by asking our patients their birth dates. But the 12 different areas of life in both systems have certain surprising similarities. The fact that human characteristics reveal themselves in different ways but with features that can roughly be summarized in 12 categories in both acupuncture and astrology has always added greater depth to my understanding of the elements. In a way, this is a comforting reminder that there really is nothing new under the sun. And my deeper understanding of the psychological relevance of what a study of astrology shows us came originally from these four books of Dr Adler.

Of course, there is also a branch of acupuncture which relies heavily upon Chinese astrology, something I know little about, but which represents another diagnostic tool used by acupuncturists.

I treasure deeply two things Dr Adler taught me. He said that each of us owes it to the world to pass on whatever we have learnt so that we can give others the opportunity to learn from us in turn, even though we may never know where our thoughts land and whose lives they will enrich.

There is one phrase of his which has echoed for me down the years (in German, but I will translate it). 'What would have happened if Mozart had not written down his music?' And Mozart, we must remember, died a pauper with no idea that his work would resonate for millions in future generations. This gave me, and still gives me, the impetus, and almost the duty, to write and to continue writing, in the belief that what I write may help somebody somewhere learn in turn from what I have learnt from life. We all owe it to others to hand down whatever thoughts we have had in whatever medium – blogs such as this one, novels, poems, paintings, music, sculpture. Only in this way will we help preserve for future generations what is valuable in human culture. And however insignificant we feel our contributions may be, we should still find the courage to make our thoughts public in the hope that they may contribute something to the lives of others.

The second, more esoteric, lesson I learnt was Dr Adler's insistence that if we cannot find something we have lost, however hard we search, then that object has really disappeared and will not allow itself to be found. We must then try to put it from our mind because it will reappear at some point in the future when the time is right and usually at quite an unexpected time and in quite an unexpected place. I have put this to the test numerous times, and it does appear to be true. I remember once frantically looking for something in a room where I knew I had last put it, only to find it two weeks later in a room I rarely used, right at the back of a drawer I would have sworn I had never opened. I also found my house keys at the bottom of the dustbin after losing them for a few days! In both cases I had no recollection whatsoever of putting the things where I found them. Now if I lose something, I just wait, and usually, but not always, it reappears in an unexpected way, long after I have given up searching for it. Try this. You may find that Dr Adler was right.

◇◇◇◇◇◇◇◇

# 2 APRIL 2015

## 'Step off into the blank of your mind'

I love this quote which comes from a poem by somebody I've only just heard about called Richard Wilbur:

> As a queen sits down, knowing that a chair will be there
> As a general raises his hand and is given the field-glasses,
> Step off assuredly into the blank of your mind.
> Something will come to you.

It represents very accurately what I often feel as I sit, pen in hand, waiting for some thought to come to me which I think is worth pursuing. At the moment, I am indeed faced with the 'blank of my mind' in relationship to writing about acupuncture. I have concluded that this may be because I am just about to set off for my seventh visit to China, and as usual my mind is preoccupied with planning what I will take with me, and, much more importantly than any clothes, what the overall aim of my time there will be. I always like to think of a theme around which I weave what we will be doing there. Last time it was the importance of developing a good patient/practitioner relationship. This time I note that I have written something about it 'requires patience to be a five element practitioner'. This echoes one of my constantly repeated mantras: 'Don't hurry. Don't worry.'

We live in a world which is obsessed with results, so that we feel pressurized 'to get things right'. In five element terms, this means 'getting the element right'. But we need to lose some of our fear of not getting things immediately right. Today on the radio I heard a well-known headmaster, Anthony Seldon, saying that everybody is now concentrating far too much of their attention on children's exam results.

Instead, we should be looking at things differently. 'Don't ask how intelligent a child is,' he said. 'Ask instead how is this child intelligent?' This is an important distinction, which also applies to acupuncture. We should not be thinking of the disease or condition that a patient comes to us for help with, but of the patient who is suffering from this condition. This is a crucial distinction which distinguishes us as five element acupuncturists from Western medical practitioners. It is not simply enough to say that a patient is of the Earth element, much as a patient, in Western terms, could be said to be suffering from arthritis. Instead, we should be thinking not about the arthritis but about the patient – not what is the patient suffering from, but who is the patient who is doing the suffering.

This crucial distinction emphasizes the uniqueness of each patient, rather than the common nature of the disease they are suffering from. We are not trying to lump a group of patients together under the heading of arthritis, or, in five element terms, under the heading of the Earth element, but instead are trying to see the patient as a unique example of the Earth element, requiring a unique approach to the treatment we will be offering, whilst still under the umbrella of the Earth element.

These thoughts have just come to me as I sit here pondering on my theme for the week in China. For a few moments, then, I 'stepped off into the blank of my mind', as the poet says, and something did indeed 'come to me'.

◇◇◇◇◇◇◇◇◇

# 3 APRIL 2015
## *'The lost art of exchanging glances'*

I am delighted to have found myself only yesterday in very exalted company, with none other than the historian Simon Schama as my companion. In an article in *The Guardian* as part of the launch of a new exhibition at the National Portrait Gallery here in London, called *The Face of Britain*, he says: '...society would be a better place if people, perhaps on their daily commute, actually looked at the faces of strangers.' Anybody who has read my blogs of 23 February and 1 March will know how warmly I support what he says.

He is also very scathing about the craze for those instant self-portraits we know of as selfies (horrible word, I always think). He says:

> What we love about selfies and phones is that it's of the moment, but the true object of art is endurance... The meteorite shower of images that we contribute to and come to us every single day in every medium, especially social media, is the equivalent of white noise, and great portraits deliver the music.

It is very comforting that I am not alone in thinking thoughts such as these.

◇◇◇◇◇◇◇◇

# 3 APRIL 2015
## *The three levels of the human being: Body, mind and spirit*

I remember one very important day during my training under JR Worsley at Leamington 30 years ago. We were learning about Aggressive Energy, and JR was explaining to us why it was so essential to insert the needles very shallowly into the Associated Effect Points on the back (back shu points) so that each needle barely penetrated the skin. What I remember most clearly was the diagram he drew to illustrate this, simply a small block of three parallel lines one above the other, with a needle just nicking the top line but not penetrating below to the other two lines. He said that this illustrated the three levels of body, mind and spirit. The superficial level was represented by the line at the top into which the needle was inserted. The bottom line was the level of the spirit, and the line between these two represented the mind, the intermediary between the body on the surface and the spirit in the depths. For the purposes of the AE drain, the needle inserted at the physical level would draw any Aggressive Energy from the spirit up through the intermediary, the mental level, and then out from the body, the physical level, at the top. This would appear as red markings around the needle as the Aggressive Energy drained away slowly to the outside air. If the needle was inserted too deeply, any Aggressive Energy was pushed further inside, causing greater harm as it invaded the spirit.

This picture of the three levels of the human being has stayed with me since then, providing an excellent illustration of the emphasis in five element acupuncture on the importance of treating the deep (the spirit) and through this also treating the physical. Many therapies, including different branches of acupuncture, concentrate treatment at the superficial level, the physical, and ignore its connections with what lies deep within us. But the two levels, with the mental acting as intermediary between them, cannot be detached from one another in this way. If we ignore the deep, it will call out more and more insistently for our attention, often doing this through the increased severity of physical symptoms. We ignore at our peril what is deep within us, our souls, and do our patients a grave disservice if we concentrate too much of our treatment on the superficial.

This is what I want to talk about to the 80 or more acupuncturists who will be gathered together at our seminar in Nanning in ten days' time. And as I have found during my six other visits there, this is one of the most important lessons that five element acupuncture can teach them.

To understand what lies deep within a patient's spirit also demands compassion from us as practitioners. Only with compassion can patients allow themselves to open up this deepest, and thus most vulnerable, part of themselves, their soul.

◇◇◇◇◇◇◇◇◇

## 25 APRIL 2015
### 'The truth is always kept in a far place'

Somebody, I don't remember who now, gave me this lovely quotation which haunts me, though I'm not sure exactly what it means: 'The truth is always kept in a far place.' The words have a lovely ring to them, and awaken in me an image of a far-distant land with, at its centre, a lovely picture of

Truth, whom I see as a graceful woman presiding over this far country. Perhaps the reason the words affect me so much now has something to do with my latest visit to a far-distant land, that of China, for my seventh visit there a week or so ago, though why should I be thinking of truth residing there?

Probably, this is because in some ways it is truth which I discover each time I return there, the truth of what I have dedicated the second half of my life to, this discipline of mine called five element acupuncture. For each visit strengthens my conviction of the deep truths about the human condition underlying what I do. Somehow in China these truths become ever more evident to me, because of the speed at which my Chinese students so quickly understand what I teach them and unquestioningly accept the fundamentals of five element practice as though they are absolutely self-evident to them. It is rare for those I have taught in the UK and Europe to reach such an instinctive and profound understanding as rapidly as do the Chinese. To us Europeans they are at first in what seems to be a foreign language, which it takes us much time to understand, whilst to the Chinese they are familiar concepts underlying all their lives.

I have been privileged to be invited by Professor Liu Lihong into this (geographically) 'far place' in a way which still surprises me for its rightness at this stage of my life. Each visit to China strengthens my bonds to my students over there and reinforces my gratitude for being given such a gift.

To Liu Lihong and the 80 students who sat enthralled in our classes as they gained insights into something which for them is often a new discipline of acupuncture, I send my thanks for the happy time we spent together. And these thanks I also pass on to Long Mei and Guy Caplan who shared this seventh step on my journey to China so creatively with me.

I am sure I heard this quotation from somebody whilst I was in China last November. Perhaps one of those reading this blog over there will tell me who it was.

# 30 APRIL 2015

## *Cutting diagnostic corners in China*

When we were students, we were always being told that we must allow our patients plenty of time to get to know us as practitioners so that they feel safe to start talking honestly about the problems they face in life and the help that they are really asking for. This is particularly so during our first interaction with them, which we call a Traditional Diagnosis (TD), to distinguish it from a purely Western medical diagnosis, something we were told never to hurry through. It is therefore ironic that, in China, time is the one thing we cannot ask for, since we are only there for a few days, and in those few days we are expected to achieve so much. Indeed, it makes me sad sometimes to think how privileged our students at SOFEA were in the amount of individual time we dedicated to each of them – individual tutorials, individual supervision of their treatments – as much individual time as we felt each student needed.

If I compare this now to what we have to do in China, I am amazed that we have achieved so much based upon the little time we have to offer anything in the nature of individual tuition to the many, many students who crowd into our courses. Nowhere am I more aware of this than in our efforts to offer each student a diagnosis of their own element as a foundation on which to build their future practice. In England, students carrying out a diagnosis are expected to spend up to two hours completing this, during which they cover a long list of questions about a patient's physical and emotional issues, with the emphasis above all on establishing a good relationship with the patient. But how do we condense this into what we want to offer our Chinese students, the 40–50 new ones coming to each seminar we give?

At first I thought that there was no way we could do this, but I quickly realized how disappointed students were if we gave them no indication whatsoever of what their own element might be. This started to have a negative effect on our teaching. We would be helping them learn to diagnose the elements of the patients brought before the class, but then were doing nothing to give them any indication of their own. And anybody who has been reading my blogs will know that I emphasize the importance of a practitioner understanding how their own element may be affecting the way they treat. So we had to think of a different form of diagnosis to fit the very specific situation we were faced with.

After a few hit-and-miss attempts at devising a way of carrying out diagnoses on as many students as possible in the extremely short time available, we now dedicate a very specific amount of time at each seminar to diagnosing, or at least attempting to diagnose, any new students coming to these seminars, as well as checking on those previously diagnosed to see whether we still agree with our original diagnosis. If we don't, which of course happens, we are quite open about telling the group that we have changed our minds (or, more specifically, our senses have changed our minds!). At the latest seminar a few weeks ago, we diagnosed 45 practitioners in one morning, a feat which required much concentrated attention from Mei, Guy and me.

Although this is a cautionary tale of just how *not* to carry out a TD, I realize that increasingly we have become surprisingly efficient at seeing the elements in this highly pressurized situation. We ask students to sit in groups of five in front of the class, each of them talking a little about anything they want to, and the three of us, Mei, Guy and me, observing them carefully. After all five have spoken, we put our heads together and come up with what we call a provisional diagnosis, one that we tell them we may well change as the seminar progresses and we have more time to look at them. It is interesting how the placing of one person next to the other often reveals very clearly their differences, showing up their elements by comparison with each other. And we have become better and better at seeing these differences, and attributing them to one or other element.

To reinforce our diagnosis, each student is then given their first five element treatment by another participant (all of whom are qualified acupuncturists). This consists of the Aggressive Energy drain (or, if we think this is necessary, the Dragons treatment followed by an AE drain), and finishes with the source points of the element we have diagnosed. And then we continue to observe them carefully in class over the next few days to see whether we feel that our original diagnosis is confirmed, or not, and in particular whether it is corroborated by the effects of treatment.

This is *not*, I repeat *not*, how a five element diagnosis should be carried out – far from it. But needs must, as they say. I would, however, beg all five element practitioners not to skimp on the time they spend on carrying out a TD just because they are reading here what we have to do in China. If only we had the amount of time to give our 45 new students which our patients in the UK are so lucky to be given!

◇◇◇◇◇◇◇◇◇

# 24 MAY 2015
## *The legacy we leave behind*

Every time I go to China I am reminded of how important the Chinese regard the transmission of knowledge from generation to generation. For there on the wall in the centre where we teach I find a photo of JR Worsley, and hanging next to it one of me, then of Mei and of Guy. Our hosts regard us as the guardians of an inheritance of traditional acupuncture which is now no longer part of the traditional medicine practised in China, and all the more lamented for its absence. And we, as inheritors of this tradition, are therefore warmly welcomed and deeply revered.

Here in the UK, and I suspect in the West in general, it is rare for such reverence to be accorded to those, like me, who have many years' practical experience. I am made aware of this each time I return from China, when I compare the number of practitioners wishing to learn personally from me, a very small group now, with the many who crowd into our twice-yearly seminars in China. What is there about us in the West that we appear to be somewhat arrogant about how much we know and somewhat indifferent to how much we really still need to learn, whilst to the Chinese the acquisition of knowledge is a much sought-after privilege?

I am also increasingly worried when I notice how few five element acupuncturists there are here in the West (and by implication also therefore in the future in China) who are prepared to go out and teach what they have learnt, something I find myself repeatedly pointing out. And here I am talking only about those acupuncturists whose five element practice is not altered by the introduction of TCM concepts, as occurs unhappily nowadays all too often. I am also concerned about how much of what I have learnt I will in turn pass on as my own personal transmission of this legacy. Am I doing enough myself?

I always remember what a very wise old Austrian astrologer and musician, Dr Oskar Adler, wrote. He said that we each have a duty to leave behind for others whatever we have ourselves learnt, however small and insignificant in our own eyes this might appear. So I am always alert to the need to encourage any who are now practising five element acupuncture to have the courage to hand on whatever they have learnt to those coming after them. There are, unfortunately, so few who want to do this, probably because they think they have to emulate JR Worsley, who would diagnose people's elements within a few minutes of meeting them. Most of us know that it will take much, much longer to diagnose the elements. This has never worried me. As JR always reminded us, 'I have been doing this for more than 40 years. You will be able to do the same when you have practised as long as I have.'

In the meantime, I try to encourage experienced five element acupuncturists to take their courage in their hands and think about teaching others. In my case, I only dared to start doing this because I was asked to run an evening class on acupuncture. At first I was reluctant to accept this challenge, since I had only just qualified, but as JR told me later when I discussed my doubts with him, 'Remember, you know more than they do!' And another tutor of mine reinforced this by telling me, 'When you teach, never pretend you know more than you do. If you are honest and say that you don't know the answer to a student's question, tell them so and they will respect you for that.' I myself never believe those who always seem to find an answer to everything, whilst I do believe those who tell me they don't know what the answer is. These I trust for their honesty.

So to any five element acupuncturist out there keen to pass on their knowledge to those with less experience than they have, I say, 'Please do so, whatever your doubts. After all, we badly need you.'

◇◇◇◇◇◇◇◇◇

# 25 MAY 2015
## *Getting to know our patients*

If you are going to be of any help at all to another human being, as we as acupuncturists surely hope to be, then we have to make every effort to get to know who the person is who is coming to us for help. And getting to know somebody is certainly not as easy as it may sound. For each of us can present different faces to the world, having learnt during our life to adapt ourselves to the different people we encounter. The practice room represents an unknown world, and at first patients will be unsure both about the treatment being offered and the person offering this treatment. Practitioners, too, meeting an unfamiliar person, will have their own concerns to face in adapting to what is to them also a new situation.

All this represents different kinds of challenges. Patients are being asked to reveal something of themselves to a stranger about whose capacity for empathy and ability to put them at their ease they are initially unsure. They will be asking themselves whether the practitioner is a safe person to whom to show any vulnerabilities, those which all of us may wish to hide from others, but which reveal the true nature of why we are seeking help. The practitioner, too, will be trying to adapt to the many different ways patients present themselves in the unfamiliar situation they find themselves in.

There is a great skill in helping a patient overcome their natural reticence at opening themselves up to another person. We have to learn ways of convincing our patients that we are a safe repository for self-exposure of this kind. We need to know what kind of a relationship with their practitioner our patients feels comfortable with, since for each person this differs. Some, with a trust in human nature, will assume that anybody in the guise of practitioner will be worthy of this trust. Others, at the other end of the spectrum, will take much longer and request much greater evidence from their practitioner that the practice room is a safe place before lowering their defences.

The initial encounters between patient and practitioner are therefore delicate affairs, requiring great sensitivity on the practitioner's part to all the little signs we give out indicating where others must tread warily when they approach us. If practitioners do not pick up such signals, we are very likely to act too clumsily and effectively silence our patient. Here, as with all things, a knowledge of the elements comes to the practitioner's aid. For each element demands a different approach from us. And as we get better and better at analyzing the complex nature of each approach, this will give us increased insight into what may well be our patient's element.

◇◇◇◇◇◇◇◇

## 25 MAY 2015
### *An amusing confirmation of my diagnostic skills*

As many of you know, I enjoy watching sport on TV, as much for the sport itself as for another way of observing the elements revealing themselves under stress. And ever since I was a young child, in quarantine for six weeks with scarlet fever, and forced to amuse myself with the only thing available all those years ago, which was the radio (of course, then called the 'wireless'), I have enjoyed listening to cricket commentaries and now watching cricket on TV. So imagine my delight when yesterday I heard a commentator describe one of the cricketers, Joe Root, whom I had already diagnosed as definitely being Fire, with the words 'Root is the heartbeat of the side.'

How nice to know that the elements evoke universal echoes in all of us, not just in those who learn about them as part of their acupuncture training.

If you want to see Joe Root in action, those of you who are from the cricket-loving and cricket-playing countries of the old British Commonwealth, look him up on YouTube, and you will see Fire blazing away.

◇◇◇◇◇◇◇◇◇

## 26 MAY 2015
### *Beware of becoming too comfortable in our work*

All of us five element acupuncturists can fall into bad habits over the years, risking becoming careless in what we do. One such pitfall is that we may become a little bit too comfortable in our work, not challenging ourselves as much as we should do. We may start to forget that each time we see our patient we see a slightly different person who is altered by the passage of time. The patient before us is not the same person we saw at the last treatment. We have to understand the need to see them with fresh eyes, requiring possibly a different approach from us.

It is indeed very difficult to retain a freshness of approach to our patients if they have been coming to us for a long time. Often we are only too pleased to welcome patients we think are doing well, because we feel they are unlikely to challenge us by presenting us with new problems. These are patients whose treatment we assume to know in advance. Here we can be at risk of falling into rather too well-worn a rut if we are not careful, thinking that our patients will be as they were before. Perhaps unconsciously, we ignore the possibility that they may have changed in some way, since changes require us to make more effort. It is much easier, we may think, to continue doing what we have done so apparently satisfactorily before.

And then we may not see, or choose not to see, something in our patient which should be pointing us in a new direction. A long-term patient of mine, whose treatment I regarded as being simple to plan ahead for, turned up for one appointment not as I expected her to be. If I had not been alert, I could easily have overlooked the slight change I perceived in her. She herself volunteered nothing until I probed a little more and discovered that quite a disturbing event had happened to her, which totally changed the direction of the treatment I was intending to give. Looking back on this afterwards, I realized that I had been in danger of assuming in advance that I would find her as I had done before, and might perhaps have ignored the pointer alerting me to a need to re-evaluate the treatment I was intending to give her, which was now no longer appropriate. We must never assume that we know our patient's needs of today, since yesterday may have changed them.

◇◇◇◇◇◇◇◇

# 27 MAY 2015
## *How quickly Metal makes decisions*

Although Wood is the element which controls decision making, it is Metal which is the best element at making quick decisions. It wants to make them all by itself, with no interference from anybody else.

It is therefore a good element to give advice, because its advice is done in short, sharp sentences, and, like any metal object, cuts straight through to the heart of the problem.

◇◇◇◇◇◇◇◇

# 4 JUNE 2015
## *The truth at the heart of five element acupuncture*

One thing I am absolutely convinced of, and was from the very first day I was introduced to the elements through my own treatment, is that there are different aspects of our life force which make unique individuals of each one of us, and that these have been given, by the ancient Chinese, the symbolic names of what are called the five elements – Wood, Fire, Earth, Metal and Water. These different aspects create our life, and, by some esoteric miracle of comprehension by these same ancient Chinese, they were understood to have perceptible presences in each of us, so that we can hear them with our ears, see them with our eyes, smell them with our noses and feel them through our emotional sensors, provided these ears, eyes, noses and emotional sensors have trained themselves to do this.

There is thus a truth underlying my practice of five element acupuncture which is confirmed each day I spend simply observing my fellow human beings and myself, and each day I practise. After all these 30 or more years of my acquaintance with the elements, I remain as fascinated by them as I was on that very first day at acupuncture college, and am in ever-growing awe of those early practitioners who perceived this truth and passed it on down the centuries and across the oceans to me, happening to sit at a party here in London next to a five element acupuncturist. As I now book my flight for my next visit to China in the autumn, I feel how extraordinary it is that the journey of my own life is playing itself out in terms of these same elements, and how fortunate I am to be part of the great route of transmission from those olden days hidden deep in the past to the present day. I am privileged to allow this small needle of mine, held in my hand as I practise, to draw to itself some of this understanding and pass it on through the tiniest of manipulations to those who come to me for help.

◇◇◇◇◇◇◇◇

# 9 JUNE 2015
## *Heartening email from a five element student in China*

I love hearing how my Chinese students are progressing in their five element practice, so I was very happy to receive the following email from one of them:

> Practising five element acupuncture these days, I got some feelings that I would like to share with you.
>
> Now, more and more I feel that it needs love and patience, just like growing flower; we just need to water and add fertilizer, then wait for it to blossom. We wait for five elements to blossom, wait for the blossom of every single life.
>
> And for a period of time, I put too much emphasis on the diagnosis of the element, and neglected building connection and relationship with

my patients, only until one of the patient gave me some feedback that I realize it.

So I calm myself down to listen, giving every patient as much time as can be, to let them express themselves. One of the patients has already received five element acupuncture treatments for half a year, but the effect is not quite pleasing. Till recently I open up myself, she said that she finds it difficult to express her sorrow and sufferings to other people, but she can pour forth to me. Afterwards, she sent me message telling me that she feels much better every time, on the second day after treatment.

How well this practitioner expresses what lies at the heart of five element practice.

◇◇◇◇◇◇◇◇

# 19 JUNE 2015
## *Curiosity – a five element acupuncturist's most important quality*

I have always maintained that one of the qualities we must develop in ourselves as five element acupuncturists is being curious about other people (and about ourselves). Without this, we will never be able to help our patients. A lack of curiosity is evidence that we are not really looking at them with the depth of interest we need to have to see them as they are.

I was glad to have my belief in the importance of this quality confirmed by something I read in the newspaper today. A reader wrote the following:

There are many reasons why we should cherish Albert Einstein. What a pity then that biographer Steven Gimbel (about whose book there was a review in *The Guardian* on 13 June) omitted one of the greatest: curiosity. Einstein is quoted as referring to this important disposition on several occasions, asserting: 'I have no special talent. I am only passionately curious.' Perhaps it was curiosity that led this patent clerk to become such a great physicist, and perhaps it is curiosity that our schools should cherish, rather than testing and league tables. (Quoted from *The Guardian* readers' letter page, 19 June)

Oh, how I agree with that! Perhaps I, too, have 'no special talent'. But I am certainly 'passionately curious. And it is this curiosity which leads me to explore ever more deeply the world of the elements within each of us.

◇◇◇◇◇◇◇◇

# 24 JUNE 2015
## *Decision fatigue*

Each element is subject to its own stresses. Mine relate to the functions of the Small Intestine within the Fire element. We know that its task is to protect the Heart, its close companion, by making sure that it only allows the pure through. This involves the never-ending work of screening everything coming to it before it allowing it to pass. Physically, of course, this means its work in filtering out impurities in the blood, but at the deeper level, which acupuncture recognizes, it also filters all that relates to our thoughts and emotions.

The Small Intestine has constantly to ask itself, 'Is this the right way to do this?', 'Is this the right thing to do?', 'Is this how I should be feeling?' This is demanding work, and just as surely as we can become too tired to walk another step, so my Small Intestine can grind almost to a halt after a day of such constant activity. It is as though I succumb to decision fatigue, lacking the strength to work out what I need to advise my Heart to do. If I am not careful, this is when I may start to do the most inappropriate things, say the most inappropriate things, send off an intemperate email by mistake, or make a sudden decision based on ill-founded reasons. With the years, I have grown better at recognizing the early signs of this tiredness, and have learnt that I need to put all my thoughts on hold until my Small Intestine has had time to recover. I have also learnt never to press the Send button on a difficult email until I have slept on it and woken to a refreshed Small Intestine, now able to resume its tasks and thus more likely to make the right decisions.

◇◇◇◇◇◇◇◇

# 1 JULY 2015
## *Treatment of a case of severe psoriasis*

I am always happy to receive confirmation from my practice that the simplest of treatments is the most effective. So many acupuncturists complicate their treatments by selecting all kinds of complex combinations of points, when, as I always say, the mantra 'the simpler the better' always holds good in five element acupuncture.

So, with my patient's permission, I am giving below the points I used for the first seven treatments of a patient who came to me with severe psoriasis all over her body, and who is now, some three months later, almost completely symptom-free. When I first saw her, the whole of her body was covered with large bright-red psoriatic patches of skin. When I saw her this week, these patches were now normal skin-coloured outlines still faintly visible against the remainder of healthy skin, so that where, before, the eye was shocked by all these violent blood-red patches, now they have faded over the whole body. Much of the upper body is completely restored to health, another confirmation, if confirmation is needed, that the Law of Cure which we all learned about at college is indeed true. Impurities do leave the body from the top downwards, her back and upper body being now completely free of any signs of psoriasis, and only faint, normal skin-coloured outlines remaining from the waist down. Her recovery has also been speeded up by the fact the she has been quite happy to discontinue the application of any cortisone cream which she was using on exposed parts of the body before she came to me.

So here is the treatment I gave her. I diagnosed her element from the start as being Wood, and I am still happy with this diagnosis. I applied moxa cones to each point, and used tonification needling technique (except, of course, for AE!). I have given the number of moxa cones for Bl 38 (43) in the list below, as these vary. The number of moxa cones for other points are those given in JR Worsley's well-known point location chart.

Treatment 1: No AE, GB 40, Liv 4

Treatment 2 (a week later): Bl 38 (43) (7 moxa cones), Liv 4, GB 37

Treatment 3 (a further week later): Bl 38 (43), (11 moxa cones), GB 40, Liv 3

Treatment 4 (3 weeks later: I was away in China so could not see her weekly as I would have liked): Liv/Lu block (Liv 14, Lu 1), Liv 4 (this is an energy transfer from Metal)

Treatment 5 (2 weeks later): Bl 38 (43), 7 moxas, GB 20 (no moxa because on the hair line), GB 40, Liv 3

Treatment 6 (3 weeks later): GB 25, Liv 4

Treatment 7 (3 weeks later): GV 24, GB 40, Liv 3

Because her skin is recovering so well, we have scheduled her next appointment to be in six weeks' time, but I have told her to phone me for an earlier appointment if any red psoriatic patches reappear.

Thank you, Elly, for letting me write about your treatment!

<><><><><><>

# 1 JULY 2015
## *'Music is no more than a decoration of silence'*

I have just been to a lovely series of concerts by students at the Royal Academy of Music here in London, hearing some of the most beautiful playing of music that I have heard for a long time. There was one particular young Polish pianist, Martyna Kazmierczak, who enthralled me with the joy with which she played. In her introduction to her pieces, she quoted an anonymous 15th-century composer who apparently said that, 'Music is no more than a decoration of silence.'

Somehow this resonated deeply with me, and set me thinking about my own work. It made me wonder whether the same profound thought, slightly adapted, could not also apply to what I do. Could one perhaps say that the span of human life, which can be seen as akin to a piece of music from its start, our birth, to its completion, our death, is indeed no more than a decoration of silence, an illustration of the Dao? We all emerge from the vast silence of the Dao, live the span of our life, and then disappear again into the vast silence of the Dao at our death. It feels good to me to be able to say that what I do is then no more than a 'decoration of silence', and that by my work I make the silence of the Dao within each of my patients slightly deeper and slightly more pure.

◇◇◇◇◇◇◇◇

# 8 JULY 2015
## *Little happy happenings*

A few days ago, as I walked to pick up my daily newspaper, a series of happy happenings occurred which made my day start with a smile. It was a sunny day, too, which always helps.

First I met an old man whose path has crossed with mine before, but with whom I have never exchanged a word. For some reason, perhaps because of the sunny day, we both stopped, commented on the weather and then passed on, wishing each other a good day. Then I walked past the window of a local café and was greeted by a waitress I don't remember having seen before, who smiled at me and mouthed a 'good morning'. I then met a lady carrying a large bowl of strawberries, obviously meant for some festivities, which, on being asked, turned out to be food for a concert to be given by Royal Academy of Music students at the local parish church. By chance I was heading to the Royal Academy, too, with a letter to the pianist I mentioned in my last blog (1 July), enclosing a copy of the blog, to thank her for giving me such pleasure at hearing her play. And finally, as I walked back home, several people returned my smiles, as though we were all happy to be alive on such a pleasant Sunday morning.

These very brief happy encounters illuminated my day for a surprisingly long time.

◇◇◇◇◇◇◇◇

## 8 JULY 2015
### *When words are not enough*

A reader of my blog asked me to explain one of the quotations with which I like to litter this blog. This was the line from a book by Elizabeth von Arnim in which she wrote, 'With this thing of chiffon she tried to protect herself from the eternities.' What did I think this meant? I did not know how to answer her, because I couldn't myself put into words what I felt its meaning was, or why I felt so drawn to it. This happens often to me, usually when I am reading poetry, but, as here, novels, too.

This called to mind something I read in a book on poetry by the broadcaster Clive James, himself a very good poet. He said that he often did not himself really understand what a certain line in a poem meant, but that this was part of its mystery. I, too, often don't fully understand the words I am reading, though some, those that I like to write about, resonate with something within me, as if they evoke a deeper meaning than mere words can convey. This is what the quotation my blog reader asked about does to me, as does another line, this time of poetry, which reverberates deep within me each time I read it. This is the line from a John Clare poem (see my blog of 29 January 2015): 'I am the self-consumer of my woes.'

Even though I am not sure what this means, I think that I understand it at a level deeper than words of mine can explain. And for everybody, certain poems evoke this deeper resonance, without their maybe quite understanding what this is. I like to think that these words reach us laden with some touch of the eternal.

And this also reminds me of Pascal's words, which echo within me each time I look at the night sky: 'Le silence éternel de ces espaces infinies m'effraye' (the eternal silence of these infinite spaces terrifies me). We could also call these 'eternal spaces', the Dao into which we disappear at our death, far-distant spaces which we can regard as terrifying, but also awesome and inspiring. I think that they must provide the inspiration behind all great art. For what exalts us inevitably at some level can also terrify us.

◇◇◇◇◇◇◇◇

# 12 JULY 2015
## *How to learn whilst enjoying myself*

There are many ways to learn, but for me there is none nicer than to put my feet up in front of the TV and watch sport. I have a particular affinity for cricket because of what happened in my childhood. In those days there was no TV, of course, but sport was brought to us through the radio. I succumbed to scarlet fever and had to be put in quarantine for six weeks to protect my younger brothers, because in the days before antibiotics scarlet fever was considered to be a dangerous illness. So there I was, stuck in a bedroom on my own upstairs away from all the family, and with only the radio to keep me company. As luck would have it, a famous cricket series between England and Australia was being played, and there were a lot of exciting matches to listen to. I had no idea about the subtleties of cricket which I was listening to (what was a 'silly mid-off', for example?), but I got hooked, and once hooked this interest in cricket has stayed with me all my life, to the extent that not long ago I went to my first cricket match to experience it first-hand. It was only then that I realized just how fast people bowled, and how dangerous a cricket ball could be.

For anybody reading this who may be interested in cricket, and particularly those in Australia who will be aware that we are in the midst of an Ashes series, there is a further lesson about the Fire element which my TV watching is teaching me at the moment. There has been a surprising turn-around in the fortunes of the two teams, with the English team suddenly transformed from a rather dour, inhibited group of players into a cheerful, expansive (and successful) team. And what do TV commentators, and I, too, attribute this success to? To the injection into the team of some new Fire people. As one commentator said about one of them, 'It's good to see a smile on his face.' Looking carefully at the whole team, I realized that three of its new members appear not only to be Fire, but a very outgoing kind of Fire, probably with the Three Heater as their dominant official, for they all seem to be what we could call 'the life and soul of the party', a Three Heater characteristic.

So if you can catch a few moments watching cricket on TV over the next couple of months, look out for the following cricketers for clear evidence of the exuberance of Fire: Joe Root (in particular), Mark Ward and Jos Buttler. And for Australians reading this, it is worth looking at their captain, Michael Clarke, who I think is also Fire, but a much quieter Fire, probably with its official the Heart Protector rather than the Three Heater.

Thus do I continue to learn whilst enjoying myself!

# 23 JULY 2015
## *Rats respond emotionally to acupuncture*

It's good to hear of scientific proof that acupuncture works, even if only in rats. In an article in *The Guardian* (22 July 2015), researchers in the States found that the acupuncture point St 36 reduced 'chronic stress-induced depressive and anxious behaviour in animals'.

But then we know that acupuncture reduces 'stress-induced depressive and anxious behaviour' for many other conditions, not only in animals but, much more importantly, in humans, too. And also, that it is not only St 36, but many, many other points which do this.

I wonder whether the rats used in the experiment might all have had Earth as their guardian element!

◇◇◇◇◇◇◇◇

# 28 JULY 2015
## *Wearing people down with Fire's smiles*

The trouble with being Fire is that I share Fire's burden of always needing to communicate with other people wherever I am. I can do this through speech, of course, but communicating through our eyes is just as, if not more, powerful. Yesterday the phrase 'I wear people down with my smile' occurred to me after I had passed another person in the street, and, yet again flashing a smile at them, realized that they were reluctant to engage with me, and indeed looked a bit dismayed at being asked to respond to my invitation.

Each element has its own burdens. Fire's are associated with its overwhelming need to relate to others. I must now think of those of the other elements, and will write more about this when I have done a bit more thinking. It is far easier to write about what affects our own element. Imagining oneself in the skin of another element is always more complicated, even if, like me, one has tried to do this for years.

◇◇◇◇◇◇◇◇◇

# 30 JULY 2015
## *Hot desking*

What a very odd term this is, some of my readers may say. It is one I heard for the first time a few days ago, but is apparently one used by all modern office workers. It appears that it is very common now for those working in offices to share desk space with others. Presumably, the term has something to do with keeping an office space warm for another person. Office workers are now peripatetic; they are asked to wander around each day looking for a desk on which to put their laptop and also any personal belongings they have. They stay there only as long as they need to, placing their things for safekeeping in a personal locker before leaving work.

I was told of a senior member of staff who had worked from her own office all her working life, but who now had been told that she, too, needs to take part in this daily scramble for desk space. She is appalled by this, and feels totally uprooted. Where can she put the photos of her family with which she likes to surround herself as she works? And does she have to get rid of her pot plants which she tends so lovingly each day? I wonder what the thinking behind this is, apart, presumably, to save space. If desk spaces are freed up when people are out of the office, I assume this makes it possible to cram more people into ever smaller spaces. But what may be the human cost of learning to view your office not as a place where you establish a second home (your own desk, your own things), but as a public space available to anybody? Has anybody calculated that? I wonder whether anybody has thought to measure the comparative job satisfaction of having a familiar against an unfamiliar, ever-changing place of work. Would it not be as though every day you have to search for a new home which you have to try to make your own? From a five element point of view, what does this do to office workers' Earth element, the element which so strongly wants to make every place where it rests its home?

This reminds me of a patient of mine who came to me because her ankles had suddenly swollen so badly that she could hardly walk. After enquiring carefully about what was happening when this trouble first appeared, it apparently coincided with when she was promoted and moved to an office on her own. Aware that she was Earth, and therefore, as are all Earth people, is happiest in the company of people, viewing her fellow office workers as a kind of work family who surround her, I asked her whether she liked this. It turned out that she hated working on her own in this way. With my knowledge of the Earth element prompting me, I asked whether she could move somebody else in with her. She was not sure whether this would be possible, but then, as often happens, the fates intervened. The management wanted to rearrange office space and asked her whether she minded sharing her room with two others. Of course, she agreed. Very soon after this, and with the additional help of treatment on the Earth element, the swelling on her ankles disappeared.

I always attributed the rather sudden disappearance of her symptoms to her Earth element's relief at no longer working alone. Perhaps symbolically, her swollen ankles were Earth's way of immobilizing her, trying to fix a home for her within herself when her actual office home had become too lonely for her. Once the office had returned to being a comfortable place peopled by others, it could be said that her body could now return to its normal shape, no longer needing to try to find its own stability within itself, which is one way of viewing her swollen legs. Fanciful though this might seem to some people, I don't think it is. Our physical symptoms always in some way reflect what is going on emotionally within us.

I thought of this patient today, although she came many years ago, because she is further evidence to me of how any environment we are in, office as well as home, will affect our emotional well-being, either positively or negatively. I suspect office planners rarely think of this when designing how their office spaces should be used.

◇◇◇◇◇◇◇◇

# 3 AUGUST 2015
## *We are all discoverers of hidden truths*

I have just come across the phrase 'the discovery of hidden truths' in a video of Liu Lihong, my host in China, on the website www.ClassicalChineseMedicine.org. Once he was introduced to five element acupuncture, Liu Lihong very quickly recognized that here was a hidden truth which he wanted me, as an inheritor of this lineage of acupuncture, to return to China, where up to this moment he felt it lay buried.

I love the expression 'the discovery of hidden truths', because I think it reflects something very fundamental about human nature. We can all be said to be discoverers of hidden truths, those which lie hidden within each one of us. The older I get, the more aware I become of these layers of hidden truths within me, and constantly surprise myself by the fresh discoveries about myself which life forces me to make even after all the many years of living which I trail behind me.

Today, for instance, this phrase stimulated another thought. Could all our lives be said to be lifelong attempts to discover more and more who we really are, where the 'hidden truth' of ourselves really is? Can we, indeed, ever say that we know ourselves completely? Here another quotation, this time from the Bible, springs to my mind: 'For now we see through a glass, darkly; but then face to face: now I know in part; but then shall I know even as also I am known.'

Perhaps indeed we always peer through a 'glass darkly' at life, with only occasional glimpses of all that lies within us, all these hidden truths which age reveals only slowly to us.

◇◇◇◇◇◇◇◇

# 14 AUGUST 2015
## *Worrying the well*

I have just watched an excellent and important programme on BBC TV (BBC2, 12 August 2015 – Dr Michael Mosley: *Are Health Tests Really a Good Idea?*). As its title indicates, it looked in depth at the value of some of the many tests well people undergo, and queried how far many of these were necessary. Importantly, in view of the enormous costs of providing health care for an increasingly aging population, it asked whether the vast amount of money allocated to these tests, which are overwhelmingly directed at the still well, would better be spent on treating the already ill. The conclusion by two very eminent physicians, one from the United States and the other from Britain, summed it all up beautifully. Surely, they said, it is better to direct resources at where help is needed, which is when a condition has actually revealed itself, and not spend so much on recommending tests for the well whose results are often uncertain, if not downright misleading. The case of mammograms, in particular, was examined here. It was pointed out that they often lead to needless, harmful and unnecessary interventions (a figure of 9 out of 10 misdiagnoses was given).

This is when I heard the very telling and hard-hitting phrase, which underlines exactly what I think is the wrong direction in which the machinery of health is heading, and that is that 'we are worrying the well'. Once we are given the slightest indication that there is a slight query about any test result, none of us will be able to forget this, and it will continue to haunt us. As I said in my book, *The Keepers of the Soul*:

> One of the many areas to be re-assessed is the Western reliance on statistics. The trouble with statistics is that they are illusory. They appear to be based on scientific fact, and offer scientific validity, but they have no meaning whatsoever in the individual case. If a test is said to offer a 60 per cent probability of establishing that a person is likely to suffer a heart-attack, am I in the 60 per cent category of the sick or in the 40 per cent category of the well? No-one can tell me this, but human nature being as it is, all 100 per cent of us are unlikely to sleep easily at night with such a statistic hovering over our heads. And yet we may never fall ill.

And again:

> Once in hospital hands, we often find they never let us go, for one test or another, imperfect as all tests must be, may surprisingly often yield a slightly ambiguous result which demands a different test or a further check-up later on, leaving us forever waiting for what we anticipate may be a dreaded result, as though shackled to a permanent pathological prognosis. This is a depressingly frequent occurrence, for no doctor appears to dare sign us off for fear of future repercussions.

I will leave it to the lovely British doctor in the programme to confirm what I so deeply believe in. 'We are frightening well people,' she said. And what I particularly liked was her conclusion:

> We are seeking technological solutions to existential solutions. We all have to get old, we all have to die, we all have to lose people we love. We are devoting resources to worrying the well.

It is rare for anybody in what I call this medicalized society, particularly a medical practitioner, to state this so clearly and so baldly. Modern society is in danger of adopting a mind-set which devotes too much time to searching for pathological symptoms instead of concentrating upon nurturing the valuable aspects of our life, and accepting the natural course of life, which may or may not include illness, but will inevitably conclude in death.

◇◇◇◇◇◇◇◇

# 15 AUGUST 2015
## *How sad it is…*

As I get older, leaving many years trailing behind me, I am aware that nostalgia for the past creeps up on me more frequently than it used to. There are so many things now which are different from what they were, and though some of these differences are undoubtedly good (though here I have to stop and think hard, without for the life of me being able to come up with even one example), many more appear to my aging sight to represent losses which can never be made good.

A small, apparently insignificant, but to me important, example of this is something which happens every morning. As I make my way out to pick up my newspaper and indulge in my early-morning coffee in one of the many coffee shops around here, I step over the wet pavement outside the front door of a block of flats, and exchange good morning greetings with a young woman who is busily washing down and sweeping the front step and pavement outside clear of any rubbish. She laughed when I told her that this piece of pavement is probably the only one now in the whole of London where the age-old practice of making sure that the pavements outside our houses are kept clear for passers-by by their owners still takes place. Now we leave all that to the road sweepers.

And just as we leave it to others to clear the pavements outside our houses, so we now leave many other things to others, without concerning ourselves with whether in so doing we are making others' lives harder or more unpleasant. I notice that if there is something like a cardboard box in the middle of the road, nobody crosses over to push it to the side away from the traffic. I remember my father stopping our car regularly, and getting out to remove some rubbish or a large stone to the roadside, because, he told us, 'A bicycle or motorbike might not see this when it gets dark, and come a-cropper.' The present reluctance to get involved extends to people stepping over any obstruction on the pavement, often at some inconvenience to themselves, rather than pushing it aside to the gutter. Let alone how very rare it is for somebody to lift up a bike which has fallen over, blocking the pavement.

It seems that more and more people are reluctant to put themselves out in any way, as though walking round obstacles is always preferable to removing obstacles. Is this increasingly selfishness, inattentiveness (everybody talking into their mobile phone – or taking selfies!) or a fear of litigation, in case their actions cause problems? Whatever, as they say, it seems to me to be a sad indictment of modern life that fewer and fewer people are concerned for the well-being of others and apparently more and more engrossed in their own.

But am I merely another example of an older person saying that 'things were better in the old days'?

◇◇◇◇◇◇◇◇

# 27 AUGUST 2015
## *The transmission of a five element lineage*

We are not good at lineages in this country, and we appear to have surprisingly little respect for others' expertise. In fact, most of our education system appears to be built not so much on the idea of learning from those of greater experience than us, but more on teaching students to discover things for themselves, almost as if the hard-won knowledge of those preceding them should be discarded as somehow not so relevant.

I have spent many weeks since 2011 in China, introducing five element acupuncture, to what must now be many hundreds of Chinese acupuncturists, and have learnt from these visits how much respect they show the lineage of five element acupuncture, which they view me as representing. This is why, there on the wall of the Tong You San He Centre in Nanning where I teach, I am greeted – each time with a slight sense of surprise – by a large panel of photographs, the first showing my teacher, JR Worsley, the second me and the last showing Mei Long, a student of mine, who initiated my first contacts with China through Liu Lihong, the Centre's director. Through his writing, he is the person who has done most to stimulate Chinese traditional medicine's search for its past roots.

For the Chinese, the line of transmission extending back to the Nei Jing, and on through the centuries to reach JR Worsley, then me and beyond, represents what they feel they have lost, a direct connection to the past. In the West, on the other hand, we seem to be, if not indifferent to this, then somewhat disinterested in the routes of transmission, as though we are not ourselves quite clear what lineage we are heir to. This probably stems from the fact that generally both in this country and in China there is little clarity about how to integrate the precepts of traditional medicine with modern attempts to draw acupuncture closer to Western medicine.

The display of photographs which confronts me each time I return to China has made me re-evaluate my own thoughts about the transmission of a lineage, and led me to a new appreciation of what has been transmitted to me. The way the Chinese view what I bring to them makes me more aware than before of the precious inheritance that has been passed down to me, and which the Chinese now clamour for me to pass on to them. Here I am, coming from a far-off land, the bearer of an unknown treasure, my knowledge of an acupuncture discipline which fascinates them. And, most importantly, somebody with 30 or more years' clinical experience, which is something they value particularly highly. I bring them a precious gift, the transmission of what they regard as the esoteric knowledge contained within the lineage of a particular branch of five element acupuncture handed down over the centuries from master to pupil. This has found its way through devious routes to the West and is now finding its way back to its country of origin through me, an inheritor of this lineage. It is useful to read Peter Eckman's *In the Footsteps of the Yellow Emperor* (Long River Press, 2007), as the best, and, in my view, so far the only, in-depth study to trace these routes of transmission.

In this country we often forget how precious the legacy of the past can be, tending to take this past for granted. To the modern Chinese, deprived for so many years as they have been of much of the history of traditional medicine through the traumas of the Cultural Revolution, anything which helps them trace this past is a gift to be nurtured. Even though all practitioners are brought up on rote learning the Nei Jing, they are aware that they have lost many of the connections between what is in these old texts and their practice of today. In their eyes, the branch of five element acupuncture I represent makes these connections clear to them.

To the Chinese acupuncturists that I teach, therefore, five element acupuncture embodies a spiritual tradition which they regard as lacking in much of the acupuncture now taught in China, and connects them to a past which they feel they have lost. Its emphasis on ensuring that so much attention is paid to the spirit is something they respond warmly to. It echoes what they have learnt from the Nei Jing, but is something which is ignored by the TCM they are taught in their acupuncture colleges.

To witness the joy with which they greet all the five element teaching I offer them is to raise an echo within me of a similar joy that I experienced sitting on my first day in the classroom at Leamington more than 30 years ago, and learning about the Fire element with the Heart at its centre. It seemed to me then, as it still does, and does, too, to all my Chinese students, that to base an acupuncture practice upon treatment of the elements was to state a natural truth about life. Learning from the Chinese approach to their past, I can now see more clearly than ever that I, and every other five element acupuncturist, form one link in the unending chain stretching from the earliest days of the Nei Jing down the years. This path of transmission passed to the West in the 20th century and is now coming full circle on its return to its birthplace, China, in the 21st century. This is indeed an inheritance to treasure.

◇◇◇◇◇◇◇◇◇

# 31 AUGUST 2015
## *What simple treatment can do*

It is always good to receive confirmation of how effective simple treatment can be. A friend of mine told me that her husband was feeling so ill and desperate that he could not work and could not leave the house. He had problems in breathing which several visits to hospital and several kinds of medication had not helped. Would acupuncture help him, she asked me. I referred him to a fellow five element acupuncturist, Guy Caplan.

This is what she emailed me a few days ago:

> Treatment seems to be going so well! Three treatments have not only helped his breathing problems but have changed his whole way of being in the world.

She also told me that a friend had met her husband, and said, with surprise, that he was 'smiling with his face'.

You cannot ask for more from such a few treatments. To be able to 'change the whole way of being in the world' for a patient is what all our work is about.

I asked Guy to tell me what treatments he had done so far. Here is the list:

Treatment 1: AE drain (none), Husband-Wife, VI (TH) 4, V (HP) 7

Treatment 2: IV (Ki) 24, VIII–IX (Liv/Lu) block, VI (TH) 3, V (HP) 9

Treatment 3: CV 14, VI (TH) 3, V (HP) 9

All points with moxa before needling.

As you can see, the patient is being treated on Outer Fire. As you can also see, the treatments have helped the deepest part of him, his spirit. In effect, he feels as though resuscitated (an excellent example of the effectiveness of IV (Ki) 24, Spirit Burial Ground).

This is also a lesson for practitioners not to worry too much if physical problems persist a little longer. I have no doubt at all that his physical problems will now gradually clear. If you treat the deep (the spirit), you cannot fail but treat the more superficial (the body). But, of course, this will take time. He has had his physical problems for many years.

◇◇◇◇◇◇◇◇

# 6 SEPTEMBER 2015
## *A reason to write my books*

I have just received this lovely pat on the back about my latest book, all the way from Australia:

> I just wanted to tell you how much I have loved reading *On Being a Five Element Acupuncturist*. Somehow I take more in from words on paper than words online.
>
> It's a gem – not only in terms of giving insight about diagnostic and practice skills but also I find it immensely reassuring and affirming. It's so nice to know that doubts and mistakes are normal and even useful. It can be particularly challenging over here in Australia where there are so few of us trained in five element style acupuncture.
>
> Thank you, Nora!

I am reprinting it here for two reasons. The first, obviously, is because it is lovely for me to hear that what I write is of help to others. The second is that I am delighted that I am helping five element practitioners understand that 'doubts and mistakes are normal and even useful'.

I have always liked Descartes' phrase, which is usually quoted as, 'I think, therefore I am (*cogito, ergo sum*).' But in fact I prefer its fuller, correct version: 'I doubt, therefore I think, therefore I am (*dubito, ergo cogito, ergo sum*).' The ability to doubt and therefore to be humble in our thinking is a rare gift we should all cherish in ourselves. This is particularly so, as I always say, when we are trying to track down the elements.

I could not have expressed one of the aims of why I write more succinctly and more beautifully. So thank you, too, Lucy, for this encouragement to continue writing.

◇◇◇◇◇◇◇◇◇

# 22 SEPTEMBER 2015
## *Paring away the inessential*

I was thinking whether there was one word I could use to describe the essence of an element, that which lies at its very core and defines its specific quality. And with the word 'essence', the words 'paring away the inessential' leapt to my mind, and echoed there for a long time. I recognized this as referring to the Metal element, and saw that it was appropriate that it was given to this element to be the first to formulate its own definition of its essential quality, and to offer me this glimpse of itself so clearly and succinctly. There can be no more condensed a definition of an element's most fundamental nature than this. I feel that the phrase goes to the heart of what distinguishes Metal from the other elements.

It is helpful to think what the word 'pare' means, and why this is so true of Metal. Interestingly, we usually add the word 'away' to the verb, thus to pare away. Again this points to a very interesting Metal characteristic, for to pare away is to discard, throw away, get rid of, and this is, after all, the function of the Large Intestine. To pare away is to remove the outer skin of something, such as fruit, and throw it aside to expose that part which we want to eat. This action is always done with a knife, and this is, of course, always a metal knife. One of the disposable knives in wood or a kind of ecologically acceptable plastic as an alternative to metal which now litter eating places cannot do the job properly, for they are far too blunt. Only a metal knife can peel away the outer layer sufficiently cleanly, as the element itself does in peeling away the outer, superficial surface of things to reveal the truths lying below. That is Metal's task, and when carried out in a balanced way this is what it does all the time. It forms the last stage of any process, its final reckoning, just as its season, autumn, exposes the skeletons of trees, revealing their essential nature before winter comes to cover them in frost and snow.

It is to Metal people that I find myself turning when I have a difficult decision to make, for I have found that they can sum up the essence of a situation quickly and in very few words, in effect paring away what is inessential in the situation and revealing the heart of the matter. This is always done in surprisingly few words. A Metal person when asked for their opinion about some problem is likely to say, 'Do this,' or 'Do that,' or 'I don't think that's a good idea,' and leave it at that, as though for them the subject has now been dealt with and put to one side, and they want to move on. It is as though they have removed the outer skin of whatever we are discussing, pared the inessential away, and pointed to its inner core, to what they consider its essence. I have therefore always found Metal's advice to be to the point (such a Metal phrase!), as if they are indeed handing over to me the heart of the fruit on the tip of the knife which they used to pare away its outer covering.

◇◇◇◇◇◇◇◇

# 29 SEPTEMBER 2015
## *How people make us feel*

Each day of my practice adds one more day of learning. Today's lesson came from something I observed in myself after I had been asked to look at another practitioner's patient. Together we agreed that she had been treating her on what I, too, considered to be the right element, which was Fire, but when I was thinking back on this patient the next morning, I remembered that I had remarked at the time, 'She's a rather passive person, isn't she?'

Something about what I had said jarred now with my feelings around the Fire element. Was 'passive' a word I would ever use to describe a Fire person, I wondered? That set me thinking of as many Fire people as I could, including, of course, myself. Nobody could call me passive, but then I am Inner Fire, and the Small Intestine is the most active of all the four Fire officials. But I could think of no Outer Fire person I knew either to whom the word 'passive' would fit. I then thought more carefully about something else which had struck me after seeing her. I had not felt that she was trying to give me anything – far from it. I felt instead that she was drawing me towards herself, which gave me now with hindsight the feeling I associate much more with the Earth element. She seemed to be expressing a need, as though asking something from me, rather than wanting to give me something, so much more typical of Fire. I told the practitioner of my doubts about Fire, and suggested that she should change her treatment to Earth and let me know how the patient was after a few Earth treatments.

It pleases me that I somehow could not leave things alone until I had traced my unease about the time I had spent with the patient to its source. This feeling about how we experience being in the presence of a particular element becomes ever stronger with experience, and we should always take note of it. It can be seen as a form of direct transmission to us of the essential nature of a patient's element.

If we interpret this information correctly by examining our own feelings and their response to what is coming from the patient, we are well on the way to finding the element.

I always love it when an element declares itself so firmly in this way, even giving me only a slight but clear hint of its presence. It may take me a little while to see what it is trying to tell me, but then it always certainly better late than never.

# 29 SEPTEMBER 2015
## *Graham's groan*

Today I happened to meet a young man in the street whom I hadn't seen for a number of years. I am calling him Graham, because it makes for a good title to this blog, but that is not his name. We exchanged greetings, talked for a short time and then parted. As I walked away, I found that his voice was so pronounced a groan that I laughed at myself for not having thought of him as Water before. What was interesting to me, and what taught me a little more about the Water element, was that the sound of this voice stayed with me for so long. I could still hear it echoing in my head many hours later. I almost felt that I was pursued by its groans.

What it showed me about Water was that a groaning voice, unlike any other tone of voice, has the ability to make itself felt in a very persistent way that I had not noticed before. It seems to me to be a clear reflection of Water's ability to push through whatever obstacle is in front of it.

I must listen now to some more Water voices to help me learn to recognize this quality in their voices.

◇◇◇◇◇◇◇

# 1 OCTOBER 2015
## *Two laments for the end of an era and one happy thing*

I start this blog with my laments. A little café, Stefano's, which I would pop into daily on my way to the clinic, has now closed and been taken over by what looks like a very much more upmarket place. I think I can no longer call it a café, but would describe it more as a small patisserie. And my favourite espresso has nearly doubled in price. Stefano and his Italian family seem to have been the last survivors around here of a time when small family-owned businesses ran a one-shop enterprise. Now the coffee chains, such as Starbucks, with their standardized fare, are taking over everywhere, perhaps understandably in view of the rents charged. Even this new little patisserie has other branches elsewhere in the up-and-coming areas of London.

My second lament is for the puzzling substitution in train announcements of the good old-fashioned word 'passenger' by the word 'customer'. I wonder who decided that this change was necessary. Did a group of railway executives with nothing better to do solemnly sit around a table to discuss the merits of the one word against the other? And why change it at all? When I hear 'passengers', I always thrill slightly to the thought of all those large ocean liners, like the *Queen Mary*, or indeed the *Titanic*, or people climbing aboard *The Great Western* or the *Orient Express*. When discussing the *Titanic* disaster, is anybody likely to ask, 'How many customers were lost?' The word now only reminds me of the money I paid today for my rail ticket to a much less exotic destination, Sussex.

But to relieve the slight gloom of writing about these two rather sad things, I tried to think of something good that has happened to me, and came up with quite a few examples, none more heart-warming than a little incident that occurred in the street a few days ago. There was a different *Big Issue* seller from the usual one outside my local supermarket, and I thought I recognized him from seeing him somewhere else. He smiled at me, and said, 'You may not remember me, but you're the lady who called to me to come across the street in Bond Street some time ago, so that you could buy a copy from me.' Now I recalled that this must have been over a year ago. So he had remembered this small act of kindness from all those months back. Perhaps too many people treat *Big Issue* sellers as nuisances, and walk on by, and too few as people, trying hard to put their lives together. We smiled at each other like old friends, and I walked on with my heart a little warmer.

◇◇◇◇◇◇◇◇

# 19 OCTOBER 2015
## *Being happy is healthy*

The following is an extract from an article in *What Doctors Don't Tell You* (8 October 2015)*:

> Be happy: it could save your life if
> you have a heart problem
>
> People who are happy and retain a positive attitude also have a healthier heart – and that can be the

---

* https://www.wddty.com/news/2015/10/be-happy-it-called-save-your-life-if-you-have-a-heart-problem.html.

difference between life and death for people who already have a heart condition. Positive people are living longer after they've been diagnosed with a heart condition, say researchers who tracked the health and psychological outlook of more than a thousand patients with coronary heart disease. They were more likely to be alive five years later than others who had a negative outlook or suffered from depression.

It's good to have this confirmation from Western medicine of something acupuncturists have always known. The Heart, an official of the Fire element, the element which brings us joy, must indeed be healthier the happier we are.

<><><><><><>

# 23 OCTOBER 2015
## *The elements' different relationships to other people – Part 1*

Some time ago I had the opportunity to ask several practitioners who were all of the Wood element what was important to them in terms of their interactions with others. After some discussion amongst themselves, they all agreed that what they always wanted was to 'engage' with people. Interestingly, two of the definitions given in the dictionary for the word are 'to interlock' and 'to bring troops into battle'. Engagement is making some kind of direct contact with another person, and also implies some kind of physical contact, like boxers engaging in a fight. It represents to me quite the reverse of somebody 'walking on by', which is more the action I associate with the Metal element's desire to avoid just the kind of close encounter which the word 'to engage' seems to describe. In their description of what they feel most comfortable with, this group of Wood people gave proof of their element's enjoyment of face-to-face encounters. They are at ease with meetings with other people which contain some quality of a contest. Again, we can contrast this with the encounters of another element, Fire, which lack this sense of competitiveness.

What Fire wants of its interactions with others is instead not a contest, but to set up relationships, gifts which the Heart, buried within this element, wants to offer all it encounters. The challenges which Wood offers those it meets become in Fire's hands offerings it hopes to give others, ultimately, of course, the gift of love. The warm smile with which Fire greets everybody is in itself such an offering, and if this is not responded to warmly in return, it will be viewed as a rebuff, a rejection of this gift. Often we will see Fire people persist again and again with their offerings of smiles and laughter in an attempt to draw some reaction of warmth from the other person. Wood, in the same position of being denied the engagement it looks for from another person, will simply metaphorically shrug its shoulders and move on, something Fire will find difficult to do, as it will judge the lack of response to its approaches to be a reproach to itself and will therefore try even harder to extract a response.

It is not a response of any kind which Metal wishes for. Far from this. It will view all encounters with other people as a test of its judgement. They are still challenges, as in some respects all meetings with other people are, because they demand responses from each person's elements, and in particular responses with which a guardian element feels at ease. Metal's challenge lies in the area of how accurately it assesses the value of any encounter. This assessment will also consist in evaluating its own reactions, for all that Metal does includes a high level of self-evaluation, its task being to weigh up all things, itself included, on the scales of some value they assign to them.

Metal judges itself as harshly if not more harshly than others. And to judge you have to stand back and observe as impartially as you can. So there is nothing here of the close involvement of one person with another that Fire strives for, or the challenging encounters Wood enjoys. Instead, there is always a space around Metal which it builds for itself so that it can give itself some distance from which it hopes to view things in as detached a way as possible. Of course, the degree of detachment and the amount of space depends upon the level of balance within a Metal person. The more unbalanced the Metal element is, the less it can stand back and observe as impartially as it should, and the more its judgement will then be affected.

And what about Earth and Water, then? That is for another blog.

◇◇◇◇◇◇◇◇

## 25 OCTOBER 2015

### *A patient's comments after his element was changed from Fire to Earth*

Here is what a fellow practitioner told me after changing her patient's treatment from the Fire to the Earth element. After one treatment on Earth, the patient told her that he 'felt a profound change. Something felt very different.'

I am always delighted when I receive such strong confirmation of the effects of homing in on the right element. My own patients have used different words to say the same thing, such as 'I know who I am' or 'I feel myself now'. That awareness of self that treatment helps patients to connect with is one of the most moving gifts our practice can offer them.

◇◇◇◇◇◇◇◇◇

# 29 OCTOBER 2015
## *The elements' different relationships to other people – Part 2*

In my blog of 23 October, I write about the different relationships Wood, Fire and Metal like to have with other people. Now it is the turn of Earth and Water.

There is some similarity between what these two elements want to experience in their encounters with other people, and in each case they express more of a need than we have seen with the other three elements. Both of these elements enjoy being in the midst of a group, Earth liking to be at its centre with others around it, and Water melding more into the group, each Water person like a drop of water absorbed into the great oceans of life. Earth will demand more individual attention, whereas Water is most comfortable with safety in numbers.

This picture of Earth surrounded by other people, preferably at their centre, metaphorically echoes the original five element diagram in which the other four elements circle around Earth in their midst. Water, liking to float as one with the rest of the world, is a good representation of the different qualities of these two elements. It helps us understand that each will want different things from their relationships with the people around them.

With Earth, the most important thing is that those surrounding it face towards it so that they can take careful note of what it wishes to say. It is not enough, as it is with Water, for it to disappear into the group, for then its words will not be heard and understood as they should be, an understanding which is a necessary part of its need to process its own thoughts properly. Processing is, after all, one of Earth's most important functions. It takes in, digests and then processes all that comes to it, both physically in the shape of food and mentally in the shape of thoughts. It then has to pass on what it has processed as physical food worked on by the stomach, and as mental food in terms of thoughts and words worked on by its mind, which it then invites others to hear.

I have always found it interesting to note the somewhat confusing messages Water seems always to be transmitting. On the one hand, it has this need in some way to be swallowed up in the whole, to merge itself with those around it, and, on the other, it has the quite contrasting but less overtly obvious need to rise above the masses around it, and thus to rise to the top. It is known to be the element of ambition and will-power, and just as water in nature exerts by far the strongest force when it is unleashed in storms and tsunamis, so a Water person will tend to achieve whatever it sets its mind to, often pushing aside those who stand in its way, as storm waters submerge all in their path. Its relationship to others can therefore often seem somewhat ambiguous. Appearing at ease in the company of others, it can then surprise them by pushing them aside, determinedly and often unobtrusively, in its fight to get to the top. A Water person might well be the one in an office who, perhaps to others' surprise, is offered the promotion these others had wanted and expected to be theirs.

And yet, despite this focused struggle to succeed, with little concern for how this affects others and often at their expense, it constantly seeks reassurance from those around it, to still the fears it always has, fear being its dominant emotion.

◇◇◇◇◇◇◇◇

# 5 NOVEMBER 2015
## *A reminder not to forget the basics: Windows of the Sky*

I had a salutary lesson recently in the danger of forgetting the basics of what I do. It showed me that it is unwise to ignore the principles that were drilled into me at acupuncture college all those years ago. One of these concerned when to use the points called the Windows of the Sky. We were told never to choose these points until we have given our patients at least eight treatments, because we need to be sure that a patient's energy has been strengthened sufficiently to be able to cope with their effect. As their name indicates, they are points which are there to open up a window on to a patient's life. We were warned that the light pouring into a patient's spirit as a result of opening these Windows too early on in treatment may shine too brightly for them to cope with the reality flooding in. The poet TS Eliot says this very well: 'Human kind cannot bear very much reality.'

The treatment I gave my patient this week provided me with proof of this. Unwisely, instead of waiting to complete the number of treatments we were told we should, I selected these points at the fifth treatment, thinking that since the patient had already reacted so well to his first few treatments, and, as he told me, was 'trying to see a way forward' in his life, it would be appropriate to select the Windows to help him do this. On his return for the next treatment, he told me that he had felt very depressed immediately after he had seen me, and could find no explanation for this. It was only when I reminded myself that this was just after I had done the Windows that I realized it was likely that giving this treatment too soon had had the effect we were warned about.

Gently talking this through with him, it did indeed seem as if he had been unable to cope with the insights into his life which these points had presented him with. I realized then that I should have waited a little longer to select these points.

This taught me, yet again, that we need to tread warily when using the Windows. It reminded me that I should always ensure that a patient's energy is strong enough to deal with the spiritual insights which are one of the gifts the Windows can bring when used wisely.

◇◇◇◇◇◇◇◇◇

# 5 DECEMBER 2015
## *Back from my eighth visit to China*

I'm amazed to think that I have now been eight times to China. Here I now sit back in London looking at the group photo of Liu Lihong, Mei, Guy and me, surrounded by the 90 people, practitioners and lay people alike, who spent a very happy, productive week with us, steeped in the elements, and learning how they can be used as part of an acupuncture discipline about which most of them have, until now, heard nothing at all or at least very little. Obviously, not all who come to our seminars are practitioners; some just attend because they are fascinated by the connections between five element acupuncture and what they have studied in the classics, such as the Nei Jing. But most want to use what they learn from us in their acupuncture practices, and have to decide at the end of the seminar whether they are brave enough to start incorporating what they have learnt into these practices. It takes courage to embark upon what is to them a completely new discipline. With great joy, I was told that some of them are now teaching others the basics of five element acupuncture, creating a little pyramid of five element practitioners throughout China.

As a very important part of this development, the Tong You San He centre is establishing a new Foundation in Beijing for the study of traditional Chinese medicine, with its inauguration taking place in a few days' time. One of its branches will be the study and development of five element acupuncture. I am honoured to have been asked to act as Honorary Adviser to this Foundation. Five element acupuncture is therefore spreading its Chinese wings ever wider.

◇◇◇◇◇◇◇◇

# 6 DECEMBER 2015
## *Our responses to the different elements*

At different times we all display the whole range of emotions associated with the five elements. One way of helping ourselves become more alive to the differences between these emotions is therefore to think back to any situations which have led us to experience them ourselves.

I am sure we have all at different points in our lives felt ourselves in the grip of fear (Water), longed for some understanding of what we are going through (Earth), become irritated by somebody (Wood), wanted to share our happiness with others (Fire) or retreated into ourselves to deal with some loss (Metal). At different times we will express each of these emotions reflecting reactions to the different stresses each element is being subjected to, irrespective of what our dominant element is. We will therefore have at least some inkling of the effects within us of these different emotions. If we extend this understanding to what we feel a patient of a particular element may experience as their dominant emotion, this will go some way to feeling ourselves into elements which are not our own. It requires some persistent work to do this in such a way as to give us accurate feedback, but once we recognize how much our work is enhanced by an ability to understand within ourselves the emotional responses of patients of other elements, this will be an enormous help in pinpointing the right element and therefore responding appropriately to its needs. For each element demands responses which will reassure it that we recognize what these needs are.

It is not only that we all feel more at ease in the familiar company created by our element, and therefore tend to think other people will be as well, but we also like to spread our particular emotional sphere around us by trying to draw other people into it on the assumption that this is what these other people want as much as we do. We therefore live our lives enveloped within a kind of cocoon which our particular element spreads around us, and in which we inevitably seek to draw those who approach us, since this is the emotional atmosphere we are familiar with.

It is a useful experiment for us as five element acupuncturists to observe our own interactions with others very closely to see what kind of an emotional net we spread around those we meet. We may be surprised to note, as I was, how often what we are offering others in these interactions is not in fact what they want. In normal social situations this will not matter too much as we have all become used to accommodating ourselves to whatever the people around us demand of us, and usually manage to shrug off what we find irritating. In a clinical situation, however, things are very different. We are not there to demand of our patients that they cope with approaches which disturb them, but to adapt ourselves through our knowledge of the elements to what will make them feel sufficiently comfortable to relax and be themselves. This is often the opposite of what happens in the world outside the practice room, and unfamiliar as this will be initially as we learn our craft, how successfully we manage to do this will depend upon some persistent work on our part.

◇◇◇◇◇◇◇◇◇

# 30 DECEMBER 2015
## *My year-end stock-take*

This is a little longer blog than usual as befits the final summing-up of a year.

I always see the end of a year as a time to look back at the months that have passed and to try to ft them into the pattern of my life. What, then, has 2015 brought me and taught me?

It has brought me much joy, and some sadness, from my family and friendships. It has brought me introductions to many new writers, many of these in other languages I am familiar with, such as German, and renewed my interest in writers I have enjoyed in the past. At the end of this blog I am listing some of my favourite reads of the year for anybody who, like me, is fascinated by the written word.

And what has it brought to my calling as an acupuncturist? After publishing my book, *On Being a Five Element Acupuncturist*, at the start of the year, I experienced a kind of mental blankness for some months. I missed the feeling of being compelled to write by something inside me. I continued with my blogs, but could find no central theme around which to build what might eventually become another book. I struggled with this for some time until one day a friend told me that her son, not an acupuncturist, enjoyed reading my books because they taught him to understand human beings better, and that he was looking forward to reading more about the elements. Somehow this stirred something in me to life, and I began to write odd bits and pieces, focusing on how I was developing new ways of interpreting my own reactions to the elements. I am continuing to do this, still with no particular structure in mind, but just darting here and there with my thoughts. I trust that a structure will emerge at some point, as it did with my other books, and that the different pieces that I am now writing will in some miraculous way fuse themselves together into a book form with which I will again hope to interest my lovely publishers, Singing Dragon.

Moving forward from my personal acupuncture-focused life to my more public life as a teacher, what of that? Well, increasingly this is now spent in expanding what I am doing in China. I have written before of how, much to my surprise, my work appears to have changed direction in the last few years, from an emphasis on helping five element acupuncturists in this country and Europe, to introducing it to China. Increasingly now, my task appears to be to continue adding to what I have so far achieved over there, which is a lot, indeed much, much more than I could ever have dreamt of when I first met my host, Liu Lihong, more than four years ago. There must now be some few hundred Chinese acupuncturists who have come to our seminars and are venturing to start five element practices of their own.

This year-end also brings news of the Inauguration Ceremony of a Foundation of Traditional Chinese Medicine which is being set up in Beijing, with my contribution to this enshrined for perpetuity in a lovely certificate I was honoured to receive from Liu Lihong in April stating that I am a Consultant in Five Element Acupuncture to this Foundation for a period of five years until 31 December 2019. Seeing this date on the certificate pointed me to further work that I need to do in the intervening years. By the time we reach December 2019, I will, I assume, be well past the age when I will be of practical use as a teacher over there, although possibly still be a kind of five element figurehead to be wheeled out at intervals to remind people of the long five element lineage to which I am heir.

In China, there are also moves afoot to translate more of my books (only one, my *Handbook*, is published in Mandarin). My non-English-reading students are always clamouring to read the others in Mandarin. I and my two regular companions, Mei Long and Guy Caplan, during our next planned visit to China in April 2016, will make our presence felt in Beijing to support the new Foundation there, in addition to giving our usual seminar in Nanning.

So my stock-take for 2015 has shown me much that I can personally be very happy about. It does a little to offset the news pouring in from around the globe of all the strife which human beings, alone of all the animals, seem to enjoy engaging in, and all the mostly man-made disasters bringing floods and famine to many parts of the world. I like to think, though, that what I can offer my patients, and encourage others to offer theirs, in some small way helps to contribute something important to the sum total of human happiness.

I wish all my readers a fulfilling and happy year to come when 2015 turns into 2016.

# POSTSCRIPT

Here are a few of my favourite books from my 2015 reading list (D = Detective story):

Wade Shepard: *Ghost Cities of China*

Jill Ciment: *Heroic Measures*

Tom Drury: *The End of Vandalism*

Jenny Erpenbeck: *Wörterbuch* (for my German readers)

Alexandra Fuller: *Don't Let's Go to the Dogs Tonight*

Robert Seethaler: *A Whole Life*

Elly Griffiths: *The Ghost Fields* (D)

Atul Gawande: *Being Mortal*

Ann Granger: *Dead in the Water* (D)

Kent Haruf: *Our Souls at Night*

Vaseem Khan: *The Unexpected Inheritance of Inspector Chopra* (D)

Attica Locke: *Pleasantville*

GM Malliet: *Death and the Cozy Writer* (D)

Alexander McCall Smith: *The Woman Who Walked in Sunshine*

Robert Peston: *How Do We Fix This Mess?*

Marilynne Robinson: *Gilead*

Bapsi Sidhwa: *The Crow Eaters*

WG Sebald: *Austerlitz*

Magda Szabó: *Iza's Ballad*

Anne Tyler: *Searching for Caleb*

Elizabeth Taylor: *A View of the Harbour*

Fred Vargas: *Dog Will Have this Day* (D)

Anthony Trollope: *Is He Popenjoy?*

# 2016 BLOGS

# 2 JANUARY 2016
## *Some problems of treating a patient of our own element*

Because my own guardian element is Fire, I can often be quicker at diagnosing that this is another person's element than happens with other elements, but this also gives me certain problems that these other elements don't cause me. We say that familiarity breeds contempt, but in five element terms it also breeds some confusion. What I experience as being characteristic of the Fire element can all too easily colour how I perceive those who are similarly Fire in ways which may be particular to me but not to them. I may assume too close a fit between them and me, and therefore think that they will react as I do. In other words, I may lose some of the necessary objectivity which we need to maintain if we are to help our patients. By identifying too closely with a patient I believe is Fire, I may overlook our clear differences, differences which are always there since we are all unique manifestations of whatever element is ours.

I may even misinterpret signs our patient's element is imprinting on them in favour of too close an identification with what I may only be assuming is Fire. For that is indeed one of the pitfalls confronting all five element acupuncturists, which is that we assume too casually and too quickly that there is a relationship to one element for reasons of our own, and not because our patient is displaying this element's signature. In my case, I relax whenever I think I am in the presence of Fire, for this is my familiar resting place. How comfortable it is to sink back into the well-known atmosphere surrounding the Fire element, and how seductive to me it can be rather too rapidly to assume that a warm smile or a sudden laugh is pointing to Fire, rather than being only a momentary Fire-like illumination laid upon the foundation of another element. After all, everybody of whatever element likes to smile and laugh, and maybe the smiles and laughter I see upon them are provoked by my own Fire-like approach to them. In other words, my Fire may be drawing out their Fire, whilst their dominant element may lie elsewhere.

◇◇◇◇◇◇◇◇◇

# 4 JANUARY 2016
## *The Fire element's Four Officials (Part I)*

I seem to be thinking a lot about the Fire element at the moment, so here in my next two blogs are some of my thoughts.

A few days ago, a student was asking me about the Fire element, and particularly about one of its four officials, the Three Heater (also called the Triple Burner), and that has set me thinking about what exactly the different functions of these officials are. They are obviously all part of the Fire element, which has as its centre the Heart, but what do the other officials do to help the Heart?

I have always had an image in my mind's eye when I think about the Fire element, and that is of a mediaeval castle, surrounded by a moat and battlements. These represent the Heart's outer protectors, the Three Heater and the Heart Protector, which work together and which I have named Outer Fire. The battlements have what is called a portcullis guarding its entrance from the outside world. For those not familiar with the word, a portcullis is a heavy iron or wooden barrier which is lowered down from above to cut off anyone trying to gain access over the castle's moat, and thus to protect the castle from intruders. At the very centre of the castle there is a further structure, again surrounded by its own fortification, which represents the Heart with the Small Intestine circling around it and protecting it. To these two officials I have given the name of Inner Fire.

I don't know where I got this image of a castle from. Did one of my teachers at the Leamington college describe the Fire element in these terms, or was it an image I developed for myself to understand the different functions of the four Fire officials? I know that it was already clearly imprinted on my mind by the time I started my evening classes in London soon after I qualified, so it has become a very long-standing representation of this element for me. And I find it very useful as it helps explain for me some of the differences between the two Inner and two Outer Fire officials. For each pair has a different function within the Fire element, has different characteristics, and therefore expresses itself differently within us, and needs to be treated differently with its own groups of points.

◇◇◇◇◇◇◇◇

# 4 JANUARY 2016
## *The Fire Element's Four Officials (Part II)*

Here's my second blog about the Fire element, as I look in detail at each of its officials.

Let's start with the Heart, and thus with Inner Fire, as we should always do, as it is our most important official, in five element acupuncture called the Supreme Controller. There it sits safely behind all kinds of barricades in rather lonely splendour, with only its companion official, the Small Intestine, granted close access. It is cut off from the rest of the castle to protect it, and there is no direct connection between it and Outer Fire. This is the inner sanctum of the Fire element, with the Supreme Controller, like a Lord of a Manor or an Emperor in the Forbidden City in Beijing, hidden well away from sight, and closely guarded by its yang companion, the Small Intestine.

Such is the Heart's importance that it has two further protectors, forming an outer defensive ring, the Three Heater and the Heart Protector. These I call the two Outer Fire officials. They patrol the castle's ramparts and form the outer perimeter of the Heart's defence system. The Heart Protector can be thought of as a guard always with weapons in its hands, defending the castle from attack. Its yang companion, the Three Heater, ensures that every part of this defensive structure functions harmoniously and as a single unit. These two officials are alert to any danger, and do all they can to prevent an attack upon the Heart deep within. We can interpret this emotionally as an awareness of the risks inappropriate relationships can pose. It is interesting to note how often an Outer Fire person may cross their arms across their chest when they talk to other people, a physical sign that they are trying to protect the Heart inside.

This image reveals some of the characteristics which the two Outer Fire officials show as they maintain their defensive attitude at all times. This can manifest itself as vulnerability when they are weak, as though retreating behind protective barricades. It is as if they are physically lowering the portcullis when danger threatens.

This kind of defence is quite unlike the response of the Small Intestine to pressure upon it. Since it is the closest official to the Heart, it cannot afford to retreat in this way, but has to stay in control at all times. Instead, its yang quality shows itself increasingly the more defensive it may feel inside.

It counters stress upon it more by verbal sparring and mental agility. We know that the Small Intestine's function is to sort the pure from the impure, rejecting impurities to protect the Heart. It is therefore constantly responding to whatever situation it is presented with by trying to sift from it only that which it is good to allow through.

When we are trying to distinguish the characteristics of an Inner Fire person from that of Outer Fire, this somewhat restless activity can be seen as one of its distinguishing features. The slightly puzzled look in an Inner Fire's eyes as it tries to sort out its responses to a given situation is a good clue. Outer Fire is not puzzled by life, just alert to its dangers.

I give below some of my tips for distinguishing the two sides of Fire from one another:

**Outer Fire**

- Easier than Inner Fire for people to relate to. (This reflects its time of maximum activity which is the evening, at the end of the day, as people start to relax.)

- Relaxed company, spreading warmth and joy around it.

- More articulate than Inner Fire, since it does not need constantly to sort out its thoughts.

**Inner Fire**

- More active than Outer Fire, since its time of maximum activity is around noon, when the sun's yang energy is at its height.

- More prickly than Outer Fire.

- Likes to spread warmth and joy, but is often prevented from doing this because it is concentrating more on trying to work out what needs to be done to help the Heart.

- Can look puzzled by life and remains puzzled until it has worked out a solution. Can therefore send out confusing signals which other people may find disturbing.

Despite these tips, it is not easy to distinguish the differences between these two sides of Fire. This is why we always start by treating Outer Fire for a few treatments to strengthen the Heart's defences before moving to Inner Fire if we feel we have not reached the core of a patient.

I like to think that Outer Fire asks, 'Is this person safe to love?', whilst Inner Fire asks, 'Is this person wise to love?'

Thank you, Mary, for prompting me to collect my thoughts together on the Fire element in this way.

◇◇◇◇◇◇◇◇

# 28 JANUARY 2016
## *A little bit of unexpected cheer*

I have been watching with fear as the world, which often seems never to learn from its past, hovers yet again on the brink of another financial precipice, with the rich making sure that they get richer whilst the poor only get poorer. And I can hardly bear to look at a newspaper or listen to the news because everywhere I see the desperate faces of asylum seekers risking their lives, and often losing those lives, in an attempt to escape the horrors of wars. I can understand what being a refugee is like, although at one remove, for half my family, my mother's half, was Austrian Jewish and many of them were forced to flee to this country before the Second World War, most of them escaping the concentration camps only because my English father could vouch for them.

And then I think of all those rich and influential people sitting around behind police barricades in five-star hotels in Davos, flying in and out in their private planes, to discuss from a distance what to do about the poverty in the world. And the gap between their world and the world outside seems to grow ever wider.

It is sometimes too much for me, and I have to take refuge in reading all kinds of escapist literature, my favourite being detective stories, where good always triumphs. I am particularly fond of the gentle old-fashioned English country village kind, which takes me back to the nostalgia of a simpler life, with echoes of my own childhood.

I am cheered, though, by hearing that at last this country will be doing something about the hordes of unaccompanied children who live in appalling conditions just a few miles over there in the camps in Calais, a prey to child traffickers. It seems as though one or more thousand will be allowed in. And high time too!

\* \* \*

There is a happy postscript to the blog above which I have just read in today's Guardian newspaper: 'Teachers flood Dunkirk school for refugees with aid offers.'

This is a heartening story of the school a teacher and friends have set up in the mud of a refugee camp in Dunkirk, of the success they are having in teaching the refugee children, and of the many other teachers volunteering to cross the Channel to offer their help. Hoorah, hoorah!

# 29 JANUARY 2015
## *A comparison of the thought processes of the different elements*

Each element will think in its own particular way. Metal will speedily resolve issues in its mind, cutting its way through thickets of thought which may hold up two other elements, Fire and Water. It will think things through at a measured pace, ensuring that its conclusion and the verbal expression of this conclusion have only been taken after careful consideration, with none of the sense of haste which Wood can show. This is so unlike the long dwelling upon things which Earth will need to indulge in if it is to fulfil its role as the profound processor of all thought. Wood will want to reach a conclusion rapidly, making its mind up quickly, perhaps too quickly, and sticking to its conclusion often despite evidence to the contrary. Water will be reluctant to allow anything to impede its need for its thoughts to flow, but may be hesitant in expressing these thoughts, perhaps often preferring to keep its thoughts to itself. Fire, particularly Inner Fire, with its concentrated attention to the needs of the Heart, will try to ensure that any decisions it takes are appropriate for the Heart, and are made as quickly as possible to ensure that the protective cover it gives the Heart is maintained.

A clear difference between the thought processes of Earth and Metal was revealed to me on a day when I happened to treat an Earth patient followed immediately by a Metal patient. I became aware that I was moving from a room in which a patient was almost obsessively concerned with repeating a story she had already told me several times to a room with a totally silent patient, who left it to me to start the verbal interaction between us. The comparison between the two was very stark and very illuminating, and probably gave me some of the most memorable insights into the differing qualities of the two elements. I could see that Earth needed me to listen and understand. It wanted to be heard, and would not be satisfied with simply telling me of an incident in its life, but had to repeat it several times in case I did not hear it properly. Metal, on the other hand, far from wanting me to hear the processes by which it had reached a conclusion, only wanted to impart the conclusion it had come to quietly by itself in the least number of words possible. It presented me with a complete episode, leaving unspoken the process by which it had reached this conclusion. It was interested only in the finished product. One could say it allowed its mother element, Earth, to do the preliminary processing work, whilst it waited to complete the action, to finalize the thought.

In each case, the speaker, here my patient, was demanding different things from me, the listener, and since these different demands reflected characteristics typical of each element, this could be used as another helpful pointer to a patient's element. Of course, these individual characteristics can become exaggerated the more out of balance a patient is, and less obvious the more balanced a patient is.

◇◇◇◇◇◇◇◇

# 5 FEBRUARY 2016
## *A plea for caution in using the point Heart 7: Spirit Gate*

It is always a joy for me when I have confirmation that what I have taught somebody has really taken root and is now flourishing. One of the difficult things I have had to learn as a teacher is to accept that much of what I try to pass on to others may fall on fallow ground and never produce the fruit I so much hope for it. Last weekend, though, thankfully the opposite happened. A practitioner asked me to come to her practice to help her with some of her patients. This proved to be a very satisfying day for me, and, I could feel, for her, too. She was eager to learn from my experience, and this encouraged me to pass on what I could.

There was just one thing that pulled me up short, and which she asked me to write about. For some reason which I still cannot quite fathom, she had been told during her training as a student at the old College of Traditional Acupuncture in Leamington that the first treatment should consist of the Aggressive Energy drain (good), but followed, not by the source points of the element she had chosen to start with, but by Heart 7, and this for every patient. For the life of me I can't think why this rather bizarre first treatment had become embedded in what was essentially a five element practice. Why would the first official to be treated always be the Heart?

In the good old days, when JR Worsley controlled the curriculum, we were always being told to be extremely cautious about needling the Heart. It is in many ways a sacred meridian, touching our very core, and therefore to be approached only with great care. It is for good reason that one of the few times we use it for any guardian element is as the last point in treating a Husband/Wife imbalance, the point which we call upon to restore balance at the deepest level. Apart from that, it can be used as a First Aid point for emergencies affecting the Heart, and, of course, as a command point, the source point, for patients with Inner Fire (the Heart and Small Intestine officials) as their aspect of the Fire element. Here again, though, we should be wary of over-use, and concentrate treatment more upon Small Intestine points.

So please, please, all five element practitioners reading this, direct your choice of points firmly to the element you have decided upon from the very first treatment, and leave the Heart well alone. And do at least 4–5 treatments on that element before deciding that a move to another element is called for. To help those who are rather unclear how to start their five element treatments, you can look in my *Handbook of Five Element Practice* for a detailed discussion of point selection in general and for point selection for the first few treatments in particular.

And give Heart 7 the respect it reserves.

◇◇◇◇◇◇◇◇

# 8 FEBRUARY 2016
## *Heart 7 again: Addition to*
## *my blog of 5 February*

The practitioner, Ruth Wallis, with whom I shared a happy day last week (see my blog of 5 February), has emailed me with a slight correction to what I wrote. Apparently, students were told to end the first treatment with Ht 7 rather than a source point of the element they have chosen to start with, only if they could not decide which element to choose. As she puts it, 'If I am happy with the CF then I do not use Ht 7,' adding that, 'You have at the back of your mind it's all too easy to think, "Oh it's OK not to assign a CF straight away because you can always use Ht 7 after AE."'

And therein lies the problem, and what I consider to be the mistake. This is my reply to her:

But who is 'happy with the CF' at the first treatment? That's really the problem. People are so worried about getting the 'right CF' straightaway that they don't give themselves time to address the elements and instead reach for Ht 7. You are right when you say about it being easy to grab at Ht 7 instead of looking for the element. I'm going to write a follow-up email based on what you wrote. Thanks for stimulating me!

Each treatment is there to ask a question of the elements and we must get used to gauging their responses so that they eventually guide us to the right element. Note the word 'eventually'. We should not try to model ourselves on the example of JR Worsley, who some of us will remember saying with conviction after only a few minutes with the patient that 'he/she is Wood'. He would say that we would all be as proficient as he was at diagnosing the elements if we had done the same 40 or more years he had. But few of any us have this amount of experience. I have completed some 30 years as a five element acupuncturist, and still acknowledge that I need quite a few treatments before I am ready to convince myself that I am treating the right element.

Because element diagnosis is such a rarefied skill, we should waste no time in the practice room. And by not addressing a particular element by reaching instead for Ht 7 we are doing that. The Ht 7 treatment will tell us precisely nothing about the patient's element (unless by chance they happen to be Inner Fire), and it will only defer to the next treatment what some seem to regard as the dreaded moment when they have to make up their minds and plump for one element. It is far better gradually to train ourselves not to be fearful of 'not being sure' of the element, and instead accept, as I do, that the initial absolutely necessary period of uncertainty, often extending to several weeks of treatment if not more, is a natural part of the process and not to be feared.

We should not be surprised at the difficulty of pinpointing the unique complexities of each human shaped by one particular element.

And even JR would query his own diagnosis. I remember him saying about a patient of mine, 'That's odd. I'm sure he is Earth, and yet his colour is not Earth's colour,' and he went away puzzling about that.

We should all enjoy the mysterious world which each human being opens up to us, and accept that this ultimate unknowability makes our work to fathom which element lies at the heart of each of us difficult but enthralling. And we should never be in a hurry, always remembering one of my mantras: 'Don't worry, don't hurry!' Patients don't if we don't.

◇◇◇◇◇◇◇◇◇

# 20 FEBRUARY 2016
## *Another example of the effectiveness of simple five element treatment*

I have just received an email from a five element practitioner which illustrates very neatly how effective simple treatment can be. She writes:

> I have been treating a number of youngsters recently and one particular 13-year-old girl has responded extremely well to some very simple treatments. Her GP had diagnosed her with hyperhydrosis – she was very self-conscious and anxious about her excessive sweating, especially of her head, neck and face, and this was preventing her from participating in sport at school. The GP wanted to prescribe beta-blockers

and had also suggested surgery to sever the nerves responsible(!).

I was undecided between Water and Wood CF for this young girl, but plumped for Water and treated her with AE and yin source points only. At the follow-up appointment, she reported to have had three bouts of shivering on the way home, despite not feeling cold, and slept soundly for the first time in months. That week her sweating had all but disappeared and she had enjoyed playing badminton, and was looking forward to a night out dancing at her first non-school disco. I needled yin source points again and left it at that. It came out in conversation that she had fallen badly in the past and injured her coccyx – perhaps the source of the imbalance?

How wonderful that such a simple treatment has proved to be so effective – and has hopefully prevented this young girl from becoming heavily medicated or subjected to some fairly drastic surgery.

I am feeling truly humbled and privileged to be asked to treat these people, and to have the opportunity to put your teachings into practice – the simpler, the better. Thank you for such wise words.

Thank you, too, Jo, for telling me this, and also for having the courage to stick to simple treatment.

There was one thing I queried with her. I asked her why she had used 'yin source points only', and omitted the yang source points. It turned out that she had slightly misheard what I had said about treating children less frequently and needling on the left side only, and somehow thought that meant doing the yin points only, not the yang. But the results she obtained by just addressing the yin is a further demonstration of the power of simple treatment.

◇◇◇◇◇◇◇◇

# 23 FEBRUARY 2016
## *Three lovely books to add to my reading list*

I love coming across good books, and am always very quick at putting aside others that I am not enjoying, even though I may only have read a few pages. I realize that the secret of a good book is that it teaches me something new about the human condition, and was pleased to find the following in an article about one of my favourite yet not all that well-known American writers, Elizabeth Strout, whose latest book, *My Name is Lucy Barton,* is now included in the list I keep of my favourite books. The article quotes her as saying about writing that her five novels have 'begun "always, always" with a person, and her eyes and ears are forever open to these small but striking human moments, squirreling them away for future use. "Character, I'm just interested in character," she says.' And then:

> But ever since I was young, I have seen writing as trying to help people. That sounds so corny but that's really what I see as my job – trying to open somebody's eyes just a little bit for one minute. So, yeah, there are times I think, 'This is foolish,' but I don't know that it's any more foolish than any other acts of trying to help the world.

I realize that in my own way I also like to think of my writing as trying to help the world understand human beings a little more, in my case particularly through the medium of the five elements.

And here are two further American writers to add to my list of favourite books. One is a beautiful writer of what are called graphic books, which is how they describe all types of illustrated books, from cartoons to novels. The writer, another American, called Lauren Redniss, has illuminated my last few days with her book called *Thunder and Lightning*, which is about the natural forces of nature. It is quite beautifully illustrated, with a handwritten text which intertwines itself around the illustrations so that each page becomes an interesting work of art.

And my final author recommendation today is a prize-winning book by Anthony Doerr, *All the Light We Cannot See*, about a young German soldier in the Second World War and a blind young French girl – very moving, very true and beautifully written.

◇◇◇◇◇◇◇◇◇

# 26 FEBRUARY 2016
## *Another chance encounter*

Readers of this blog know that I enjoy going to coffee houses and doing my writing and my reading over coffee. Often, too, I don't finish the cup, but just enjoy the smell and the feeling of excitement it always give me. I have traced this back to when I was a teenager, and the first coffee shop in London opened in Wigmore Street. This would be where I met an uncle who, being originally from Austria, was helping me with my German studies as I prepared for my university entrance exams. Then a second coffee shop opened in Hampstead, and again I can feel the thrill of travelling up to North London from our South London home, emerging in Hampstead High Street opposite the Everyman Cinema, and feeling myself in the heart of London's intellectual life. A coffee shop, a book and something to write with and write on therefore still remain tinged for me with the exciting aura of the past.

And I would like now to acknowledge the friendliness of all the staff at one of my favourite coffee houses, Paul's, here in Marylebone High Street. I now know each by name, and they always greet me with warmth. And, too, to my surprise, I discovered recently through a chance encounter that two people who are often here at the same time as me happen to have known this same uncle who introduced me to coffee houses all those years back. This is another example of what is called a serendipity – something that happens quite by chance, but seems somehow to be pre-ordained.

I love the word 'serendipity'.* First, for its sound which has within it a clear reference to a kind of made-up childish word I use, 'dippity', which is in not in my dictionary (although 'dippy' is, meaning 'crazy' or 'silly', and 'of uncertain 20th C origin'), and for me describes a somewhat scatty kind of a person. And this always sets me thinking on a well-worn, nostalgic path which leads directly to my mother. For I remember her well one day, a few years after I had established my acupuncture college, saying to me, 'I always wonder how a flibbertigibbet like you got it together to run a school.' So, to her, all the length of the half-century of the lives we lived together I must have remained this very scatty, dippity sort of person I certainly was as a child.

The thought of this serendipitous meeting with my uncle's acquaintances in my favourite coffee shop this morning brought this all back to me.

---

* The *Concise Oxford Dictionary* defines 'serendipity' as 'the faculty of making happy and unexpected discoveries by accident' (coined by Horace Walpole in 1854).

# I MARCH 2016

## *Theory versus practice*

I have just spent a morning listening in admiration to Elisabeth Rochat de la Vallée talking about the points I love, the Windows of the Sky. She said that these could also be called Windows of Heaven, since the character is really that of heaven, and this added another layer of meaning to the use of these points. Her knowledge of Chinese and of the ancient texts, both medical and philosophical, is very profound, probably the most profound of anybody in the world at the moment. At a theoretical, abstract level, what I learnt is fascinating, but, as always, I find that I have difficulty applying to my practice what I have been told about the symptomatic application of the various acupuncture points discussed. So much of what I learned today therefore interested me from a theoretical rather than a practical point of view.

And this is how I have tended to view what I learn from those books which list points in terms of their symptomatic importance. I always like to ask myself whether those whose texts we are referring to, both those coming from the far-distant past as well as those recently published, were or are experienced acupuncturists. What has always been a sticking point for me is how far we are able to accept that what is told us can be shown to be soundly based on practice, rather than just being anecdotal. Being the kind of person who needs to assess how far I trust the experience of those teaching me, and thus remaining sceptical until proven otherwise, I treat such recommendations with caution. It is only once I feel that somebody is basing what they are saying upon deeply felt conviction and personal experience, and shows the kind of human empathy and kindness I expect of those helping their fellow human beings, that I can add what I am being told to my own practice.

Of course, this means that there are not many people who can convince me of the validity of their level of practical experience. I have, though, been fortunate in having met some few people with deep enough experience and understanding to illuminate my path, foremost among them, of course, my teacher, JR Worsley.

In the field of acupuncture, one area which Elisabeth Rochat represents at the highest level is that which relates to pure scholarship – the ability to study an ancient language and reveal what it is telling us as accurately as possible. Quite another area is that which deals with our practice – the ability to translate what has been learnt based upon having treated a sufficiently large number of patients to pass this learning on to other practitioners. These two areas demand quite different skills, and must not be confused. A scholar steeped in ancient Chinese cannot teach me what I feel confident enough to incorporate into my daily practice, but can deepen a different level of my understanding of what I do. An experienced acupuncturist whom I respect can teach me much that will help me in my daily practice.

I think people often confuse the two.

◇◇◇◇◇◇◇◇

# 8 MARCH 2016
## *Each of our lives should make a difference*

It is lovely coming across inspiring words. The ones I have just read are from an interview with Bianca Jagger in today's *Guardian* newspaper. And if you want a good example of the Metal element, then you can also learn more about this element from her photo (I think her photo shows some of the dominant characteristics of this element quite clearly).

She has always been a great fighter against injustices wherever she finds them, a woman really to be admired. The article finishes with these words from her: 'Sometimes I say I work too much, I travel too much, I need a rest. But I'm glad that I'm doing this. I don't think I would be happy to have a life of leisure.'

The interviewer then asks her what she hopes her legacy will be. When she speaks, her eyes start to well up. 'I hope I was able to make a difference. That's all we can hope for. That I can look back and say I tried.'

We should all emulate Bianca Jagger in ensuring that some aspect of our life 'has made a difference'. This does not mean it has to make a huge or a public difference, as her life has done in many areas. The importance is for each life to have had its own moments of significance, of having made some slight difference to the world, of having changed something, however small, for the better. This is what I hope from my own life.

◇◇◇◇◇◇◇◇◇

# 1 APRIL 2016
## *Designer bicycles*

We seem to have entered the age of the 'designer' everything. There are, I am told, designer prams, much admired and sought after by the rich, with names such as a Ferrari or a Mercedes pram, and thus presumably, designed by these car manufacturers like racing cars. Not only these, but today I noticed a snazzy bike at the front of the shop window of an upmarket handbag shop. Presumably designer bikes will soon be, or are already, the next must-have for those with too much money to spend.

I remember the days when we wheeled our children in easy-foldable pushchairs which did not clutter up shops or buses as today's indecently cumbersome prams with their large wheels do. This was before the time when prams, and now bicycles apparently, demanded the attention of special designers to attract customers. I don't always think back nostalgically to the old days, but some things really did feel simpler then. Perhaps we were still so shell-shocked from the war that we were delighted just with the simple possessions available after a time of great deprivation. We certainly felt it was wrong to spend money on useless luxuries, even if these were available to us. It is these that now fill our shops.

◇◇◇◇◇◇◇◇

# 7 APRIL 2015
## 'Who would have the imagination to invent that?'

There was an interesting discussion by an award-winning Harvard mathematician on BBC *Today* programme yesterday. He was talking about the work of a mathematician from an obscure town in India, Srinivasa Ramanujan, who is the subject of a film I want to see, almost for its title alone, called *The Man Who Knew Infinity*. The person being interviewed said of Ramanujan's work: 'It must be true because who would have the imagination to invent that?' I found that a very profound thought.

'Infinity', which is in the name of the film, is another word for what we call the Dao, the All, that which lies behind and beyond all that is known, but which encompasses everything. I am always heartened when I hear of creative people who live their lives in some way constantly in touch with infinity. They are found in all areas of life, from art, to literature, to music, to theatre and film, and also, much in my mind at the moment, to architecture, now so sadly deprived of one of its most shining jewels, Zaha Hadid.

I realize that the words I heard on the radio which referred to the sphere of mathematics also in some way apply to what I do. Perhaps we 'know infinity' each day as acupuncturists when we work with the elements, and through them attempt to reach the deepest part of what it is to be human. When I feel my treatment has achieved what I want it to, I can indeed feel that the fundamental truth embodied in acupuncture must be valid because 'who would have the imagination to invent it?'

◇◇◇◇◇◇◇◇

# 11 APRIL 2016
## *The effect of needling a Window of the Sky: Heavenly Pillar*

A patient gave me this lovely description immediately after I had needled Heavenly Pillar, III (Bl) 10, the Water element's Window of the Sky:

> That was a big point. It felt like there was a trickling all the way down my spine. It was like listening to music.

So here is proof, if proof is needed, that a Window does indeed open our spirits up to what lies beyond us.

◇◇◇◇◇◇◇◇◇

# 12 APRIL 2016
## *Another good use of the moxa stick*

I am a great believer in the powers of the moxa stick for all sorts of skin conditions which don't respond well to other forms of treatment. Here is another example of this.

A 14-year-old boy had a very nasty large patch of itchy, toughened skin around his knee, about 4–5 inches (10cm) in diameter, given the name of lichen simplex chronicus, for which the specialist as usual prescribed steroid cream. I immediately produced a moxa stick, and suggested that this should be used as many times a day as possible by waving it slowly and as closely as possible over the scaley, leathery skin until the whole area was thoroughly warmed up.

Within a day, the itching, which had been unbearable before, had improved, and the skin started to look pinker and healthier. Today, three days later, I was told that the skin is beginning to look very much like back to normal. It is lucky that the boy so enjoys using the stick that he sits hunched over his knee four times a day, hence the speed with which the area is starting to regain its normal appearance.

I have always said that every home should have a moxa stick in its own moxa holder (a small candlestick of the right size can be used for this), ready to be used whenever the skin is affected in any way. Boils, cuts, psoriasis and all conditions affecting the skin can be miraculously healed in a surprisingly short time. I used it on somebody with a very large weeping blister on one of my walking tours, and was known ever after as 'the lady with the magic stick', when, even to my surprise, the blister healed sufficiently to make walking possible the next day.

It is also excellent for bedsores in bed-bound people, although hospitals are unlikely to allow it for fear of setting off the fire alarms. One very ill patient of mine, though, insisted on asking for her very painful bedsores to be treated with the stick. Surprisingly, the hospital agreed to this, perhaps because she was very close to the end of her life, and she told me triumphantly how much it had helped reduce the pain, to the nursing staff's surprise.

◇◇◇◇◇◇◇◇◇

# 27 APRIL 2016
## *Thoughts on my return from my ninth visit to China*

This blog is for all the dedicated Chinese five element acupuncturists and budding acupuncturists who came to our seminars and public lectures in Nanning and Beijing on my recent visit to China, some of whom I have taught nine times over the past five years.

So, who are they?

Well, there were 35 students in our four-day advanced seminar in Nanning. Then there were 120 more students and interested observers at a public lecture we gave at the Beijing Traditional Medicine Hospital, plus 350 or so more at a similar lecture for students at the Beijing University of Traditional Medicine.

And finally at two packed days of clinical seminars at different acupuncture clinics in our last two days in Beijing. there were 50 people on Saturday and 30 on the final Sunday. So we flew home on the Monday morning having spoken about five element acupuncture in all to nearly 600 people, as well as treating more than 30 patients in front of them on clinical days. I begin now to understand why so many copies of the Mandarin version of my *Handbook* have been snapped up in China.

All in all, a truly prodigious feat for all three of us – Mei Long, Guy Caplan and me. We shared each teaching day, with a surprising level of harmony between us, as well as a surprising degree of agreement about people's guardian elements. We have developed into a very cohesive and effective teaching unit, each with our own particular expertise. Guy concentrates on helping students with what we call their CSOE skills (those of recognizing the colour, sound, smell and emotion of the different elements). He has developed many interesting and innovative ways of teaching them how to start diagnosing the elements through their senses. Mei offers both sound clinical skills and the relief for our audiences of not needing to have to wait for each word to be translated into Chinese. I offer my 35 years' experience and whatever else is needed, often concentrating on helping students observe me in my interactions with patients as I carry out diagnoses in front of the class.

All three of us combine well in diagnosing participants' elements, something eagerly sought by all, and so essential for any five element practitioner. We have become increasingly skilled now at bringing together our different insights into the elements to form a preliminary diagnosis which is then confirmed or amended as we get to know the participants. Each person is then given a treatment, starting, of course, with an AE (Aggressive Energy) drain, and finishing with the source points of the chosen element. We are flexible, too, about amending our diagnosis if time with the students leads us to change our minds.

All this helps the students develop their own insights into the elements, as well as confirming the need to ensure that they retain the humility necessary for anyone working with the elements, to allow the elements, those elusive agents of transformation, to teach us and prevent us from becoming too fixed in our ideas about their different qualities.

I started writing this blog at Beijing Airport waiting for the flight back to London, warmed to the heart by the welcome we had received, and by the delight I personally experienced to discover how well the participants had absorbed so much of my teaching over the five years I have been visiting China. This time, for the first time, I asked those bringing patients to be treated to list the last five treatments they had given, and was pleased to find how well they had taken in all that we had taught them. This can be summed up in two of my mantras: 'The simpler the better' and 'Don't worry, don't hurry'. Their treatments were indeed simple, and focused clearly on one element at a time, and they didn't seem to worry when we changed the elements, nor did they seem to be in any hurry. Rather, they appeared to have taken to heart the need for flexibility when trying to diagnose the elements, without feeling under too much pressure 'to get it right', which has unnecessarily bedevilled much five element practice in this country.

And now I am just about to finish reading an excellent introduction by Heiner Fruehauf to the long-awaited English translation of Liu Lihong's book *Classical Chinese Medicine*, about to be published. His book, which has sold over 400,000 copies in China, has drawn attention to the need to reconnect Chinese medicine to its traditional roots to prevent it from becoming swamped, as it is at present, by the pressures upon it of Western medicine. I feel much humbled when I realize that my own efforts to return five element acupuncture to its birthplace have joined this growing current which is drawing traditional Chinese acupuncture into the mainstream of medical care in China and on into the world outside.

Part of this trend is the recent inauguration of the Beijing Tongyou Sanhe Traditional Chinese Medicine Development Foundation, under the aegis of Liu Lihong, for which I have received an impressive certificate stating that I am an adviser to the Acupuncture Committee for a period of five years.

◇◇◇◇◇◇◇◇

# 2 MAY 2016
## *A nostalgic trip into my past*

I am reading a rather delightful book I picked up by chance in the library. It is a diary by somebody called Kathleen Hey, who was a shop assistant in Yorkshire during the Second World War. It brings back very clear memories of my own childhood, particularly the four-year period we spent escaping the London Blitz to Bowness-on-Windermere in the Lake District. Opposite the small house at the lakeside, a former café, into which we crammed our large family of relatives and friends who had escaped to England from Nazi-occupied Austria, was a small, derelict refreshment kiosk to which we as children would press our noses because, displayed on its dust-covered shelves, were cardboard replicas of the sweet and chocolates now no longer available in the wartime shops.

I was reminded of the feelings of longing I had each time I passed the kiosk by what I have just read in Kathleen Hey's diary, as she describes a few days' holiday in Blackpool:

There were queues at all food shops, some serving customers (residents) at one counter and visitors at another. By the time a woman on holiday has shopped for her family the morning will be gone. There are no cigs, sweets or matches though many of the windows are attractively dressed with dummy boxes.

I still have some of this longing for chocolate which must have been sparked by the dummy boxes in the empty kiosk all those years ago. Give me a box of chocolates now and I am hard put not to finish it at one go.

Thus are we all conditioned by what happens to us in our childhood.

◇◇◇◇◇◇◇◇

## 19 MAY 2016
### *One of the many challenges of being a five element acupuncturist*

We must never be too quick to say, 'I know this patient's element is obviously Fire (or Wood or Earth or Metal or Water).' There is nothing 'obvious' at all about the way in which an element presents itself to us. We may learn to recognize its presence more and more clearly with time, but we should always keep a healthy small (or large) question mark hanging over it, reminding us that elements can hide themselves so subtly behind manifestations of other elements that they still have the power to surprise us, as they do me even after all these years.

If the presence of an element were so simple to detect, we would all be brilliant five element acupuncturists early on in our career, but human beings are much more complex than we think. So we should never underestimate the time it will take us to find the one element buried deep within the circle of all the elements which gives each of us our individual stamp of uniqueness.

Pride, as they say, comes before a fall, and never is this truer than when trying to diagnose an element. We risk much if we think our understanding of the elements is greater than it truly is.

In any case, the secret of good five element acupuncture is not simply managing to diagnose the right element, despite this being what many practitioners think. Instead, it is learning to respond appropriately to that particular element's needs. Even if we diagnose the right element, do we know how to respond to its needs in a way which makes the patient feel that they have been heard as they want to be heard? If that understanding is not there, treatment will rest on fallow ground, however much it may be focused upon the right element.

Supposing, for example, that we diagnose a patient's element, correctly, as Metal, but respond to it in a way which would be more appropriate to an Earth patient, offering a 'oh dear, oh dear, you poor thing' kind of response, we will find that our Metal patient soon backs away and decides not to continue treatment. Our element may be Earth and it may be natural for us, mistakenly, to offer to all our patients what we ourselves feel most comfortable with. Unfortunately, however, we have to learn to feel comfortable in the company of elements not our own. To surround Metal, for example, with a kind of enveloping sympathy is not what it wants. It will feel suffocated by it, its Lung unable to breathe. Instead, we must learn to offer the space it always wants to place between itself and others.

And the same holds true for how we need to approach our interactions with the other elements. As far as possible, then, we must learn to suppress the needs of our own element and think ourselves into those of the element we have chosen to treat. This is not an easy task, and one that it takes some skill and much practice to acquire.

◇◇◇◇◇◇◇◇

# 10 MAY 2016
## *Nostalgic memories*

It is strange to become aware of social change happening before my eyes as happened today. I was reading an excellent book about Shakespeare's life by James Shapiro, called *1606 – Shakespeare and the Year of Lear*. Shakespeare wrote *King Lear* around the time of the Gunpowder Plot, with Guy Fawkes one of the conspirators. For the next 400 years this day has been remembered by the fireworks displays we hold on 5 November.

But I now realize that things have changed almost without my noticing it. It must be many years since I last passed a few ragamuffins on the street pushing along an old pram in which they had stuffed a hastily dressed puppet, and calling out to me as I pass, 'A penny for the guy?' We still celebrate Guy Fawkes Day with fireworks, but children no longer re-enact the event symbolically by wheeling a model of Guy Fawkes around in an old pram. Are there indeed still any shabby old prams out there suitable for this, rather than the huge modern contraptions blocking our pavements? And pennies have long since disappeared. But I was pleased when my colleague, Guy, told me that he remembers as a child dressing his teddy bear up in old clothes, propping him up in the street and begging passers-by for pennies.

Another nod to our past has thus gone almost without our noticing it. Just as I can't remember how many years it is since I last heard groups of carol singers knocking on doors up and down the street before Christmas, although maybe this still happens in small rural communities where people know their neighbours. Some of the carol singers would gather in groups and collect for a charity, but often we would open our door to two or three young children, who would launch into feebly singing a few odd bars of 'Good King Wenceslas', before grinding to a halt because they didn't know the words. Perhaps nowadays, too, it would be considered too risky for young children to knock on doors on their own in the evening, another sad indictment of the times.

When customs such as these which have persisted for centuries lose their relevance, dwindle and die out, a little fabric of our social history is torn away with them. Now all the new customs are created, not on the streets but at one remove on social media through our mobile phones.

◇◇◇◇◇◇◇◇◇

# 15 MAY 2016
## *The power of releasing blocked energy*

I love clearing what we call energy blocks, a technique which really forms the bedrock of five element practice. All illness can be described as being caused by different forms of blocked energy, being the result of some impairment of the balanced flow of energy from element to element round the five element circle. The most common form of block, and one we address at a patient's first treatment, is that which leads to the presence of Aggressive Energy, an AE block, where one

element in distress passes its disturbed energy on along the cycle, not to its child element but to its grandchild, throwing it across the circle 'like some hot potato', we were told.

It always amazes me how many physical complaints can disappear simply by expelling this negative energy from body and soul, and how often it will occur as a result of some mental or physical trauma. Any form of surgery, for example, life-saving though it may sometimes be, must always be viewed as traumatic for the body (and soul), and therefore benefits from checking for the presence of AE afterwards. It may well be there, and will hinder recovery if left to fester for too long. In a fairly healthy person, I assume that AE will gradually seep from the body without treatment – otherwise nobody would recover from surgery or other traumas, which, of course, they do – but recovery will be speeded up if this simple treatment is done as a matter of course.

Then, of course, there are all the frequent day-to-day blocks we encounter, which we call Entry/Exit blocks, blocks which occur at the exit point of one meridian and the entry point of another. These lead to localized areas of pain and discomfort, which can speedily be dispelled by the needling of just a few points. Finally, there is the most powerful Entry/Exit block of all, that between Conception Vessel and Governor Vessel, a CV/GV (Ren Mai/Du Mai) block.

I remember JR Worsley telling us that we would do the points for a CV/GV block on every patient if only they were on the hand. I recall laughing at the time, but I have since realized how true this would be because of the wondrous power this releases at the deepest level. I suspect many of us choose not to detect this block from a natural reluctance to needle what is the most intimate part of a person's body. To help our students at SOFEA overcome their inhibitions, we always made sure that they had marked up these points on both men and women as part of their training. (And here I will pass on a tip I have learnt from Chinese acupuncturists, who

are much less reluctant to needle these points than the more inhibited English. Turn a patient on their side with their knees bent, rather than, as we were taught, needling the points with the patient lying on their back, a more vulnerable position, certainly for women.)

A patient on whom I have just needled a CV/GV block told me that she felt very different immediately after the treatment. 'I feel more centred, more grounded, more upright.'

See also my *Handbook of Five Element Practice* for more on all kinds of blocks.

◇◇◇◇◇◇◇◇

## 21 MAY 2016

*Example of why it is so satisfying*
*teaching my Chinese students*

Here is an email I have just received from one of my acupuncturist students in China, who brought several of her patients to our recent seminar for us to help diagnose and treat:

> Thank you so much for what you did to help me to diagnose my patients' elements in Nanning and Beijing. When I came back home I treated them. Almost everyone feels well, and I also see the changes in them, especially in my mother-in law. I treated her on the Metal element. She knows that she should let go more, and she is softer as a person. So now I can get on well with her.

It is so pleasing to receive such strong confirmation that what we have been teaching over in China for the past five years is falling on such productive ground. I'm so glad that this particular student of ours is now getting on better with her mother-in-law, with whom she lives. It shows how important for our relationships it can be if we work out what the elements of our nearest and dearest are. We can then allow them to express themselves in the way they need to, rather than bemoaning the fact that they don't behave as we would like them to do.

◇◇◇◇◇◇◇◇

# 15 JUNE 2016
## *Europe – in or out?*

Oh, this wretched referendum being forced on this country against our will! Who wants a referendum except those who want us to get out of the EU? Certainly, I don't, and I don't know many people who do. I have always regarded myself as European to the core, and never a Little Englander, so I fervently hope that there are more people who think like me out there voting on 23 June than those who don't.

I come of a family for whom Britain's connections to Europe dominated throughout the years of my childhood during the Second World War, and one which had suffered deeply and often tragically from the xenophobic and racial hatreds which led to the war. Unhappily, these now seem to be rearing their very unpleasant heads again, as poor suffering migrants, escaping the kind of persecutions my mother's Austrian Jewish family had to suffer, are now being made scapegoats for many of the real problems people in this country (never the rich, mind you) are suffering.

I think we are going through strange and extreme times, of which the referendum is one symptom, as are the other odd signs of this, such as Donald Trump's successes in the States, the rise of increasingly right-wing, almost fascist parties in Europe and the corresponding, and necessary, rise of parties of protest, such as those in Greece or Spain, and even what is happening to the Labour Party in this country. The political uncertainties all this creates raise disturbing echoes of those at other troubled times, most obviously in the 1930s, which led to the rise of fascism in Germany and Austria, my mother's and my birthplace.

In turn, this has been accompanied, for me personally, by a renewed interest in the tumultuous background to my earliest years during the war. By coincidence, several things have concurred to bring this period of European life to the forefront of my thoughts, among them the reading of some highly interesting books which have illuminated this period for me. First, there is the recently published book by Philippe Sands, the international lawyer, called *East West Street: On the Origins of Genocide and Crimes against Humanity*, a book of great interest not just to lawyers but to all those whose family suffered persecution under Hitler. Philippe Sands interleaves his legal discussions relating to the background to the Nuremberg trials with discoveries about the history of his own family in Nazi-occupied Poland. Coincidentally, there are connections with my own family, since Philippe bought my mother's house in Hampstead, and my mother's cousin helped him decipher and translate some of the handwritten German documents he discovered during his search for his family.

The reading of this book also coincided with a re-introduction through a friend to an Austrian writer, Ilse Aichinger, whom I remembered reading some years back but had completely forgotten about. She told me of Ilse Aichinger's only novel, called, in its first English translation, *Herod's Children,* published in its original German in 1948, with the translation appearing in 1956. This book, too, is about the period of the Second World War, and follows a group of Jewish children in Vienna whose only permitted playground is a graveyard. It is not a realistic representation of Viennese life under the Nazis, but a kind of mythical transposition viewing the world through a child's eyes. It is a book which deserves a much wider readership than it has at present. So I am now on a mission to try to interest Daunts', my favourite bookseller, to re-publish it, as it deserves to be out there again as one of the discoveries of forgotten masterpieces which they pride themselves on publishing.

Finally, to round off these few weeks of immersion in the past, I saw an amazing film called *Son of Saul,* about a Jewish prisoner in a concentration camp, who is part of the Sonderkommando, those prisoners who were set apart and given a few more months of life in order to act as guards, shepherding their fellow Jews into the gas chambers. He thinks he sees the body of his son, and the film is the story of his despairing attempts to find a Rabbi amongst the prisoners so that he can give his son a proper burial. I was persuaded to see the film only after a friend reassured me that you do not directly see any of the terrible events taking place, but as dim background to the camera's view which is trained always upon the father, particularly just on his face. It is one of the most moving and, yes, uplifting films I have seen. Go and see it if you can still catch it.

◇◇◇◇◇◇◇◇

# 27 JUNE 2016
## *The disappearance of things*

I have written before about a very interesting old Viennese musician and astrologer I knew many years ago called Dr Oskar Adler. I remembered one of the things he would say after a curious incident which happened to me yesterday. He believed that it is pointless looking for things that we have mislaid, because they really go missing. You have to leave some time, and then they will reappear.

I had further proof of this rather esoteric belief again. Anybody of my venerable age will know that the one object they treasure above all others is the old people's free bus pass, which allows us to hop on and off buses and in and out of tube trains at will, and gives us the kind of freedom denied previous generations of the elderly. I always check that I have my pass before I leave home. This morning, to my dismay, it was not where it usually is, tucked safely away in the front compartment of my rucksack. I searched for a long time for it, looking into all the pockets of all the clothing I might have been wearing on my last trip outside, but could find it nowhere.

I decided that I should immediately apply for a replacement at the local Post Office, and so headed outside to do just that. I was standing on the top step of the short flight of stairs leading to the road outside, when I happened to look down. There on the pavement, tucked closely against the front railings, was my bus pass. The road sweeper had obviously recently been, because the pavement was swept completely clean, the only object in sight on the ground being this little plastic rectangle in its white cover. If I had grasped the right-hand rather than the left-hand railings to help me down the stairs, I would have missed seeing it completely.

I still can't think how it got there. Rationally, I could say that it might have slipped from the rucksack as I got out my front-door keys the day before, but I prefer the more mysterious explanation. My bus pass decided to do one of those disappearing tricks that Dr Adler persuaded me to believe in, and simply took it in its mind to reappear on another day.

In the past, when something similar has happened to me, which it has done several times, the time between an object's disappearance and reappearance has often been longer, sometimes a few weeks. And once I found the keys to my house, for which I had desperately hunted for days, hidden away a few weeks later under rubbish at the bottom of an outside dustbin.

I like to think that there are indeed 'more things in heaven and earth, Horatio, than are dreamt of in your philosophy' (*Hamlet*). This little incident lifted my spirits a little, just a little, from despairing and dreary contemplation of the weekend's political turmoil.

◇◇◇◇◇◇◇◇◇

## 17 JULY 2016
### *A good example of the Fire element*

Here are some comments from the BBC Sports Website today about Andrew Johnston, the English golfer, a competitor at the golf tournament at Troon.

[Andrew] has delighted fans at The Open with his cheerful demeanour and says he will continue to do so when chasing the Claret Jug on Sunday.

The Englishman high-fived spectators as he walked down the 18th and his one-under 70 left him on five under, seven adrift of leader Henrik Stenson.

Playing in only his second Open, the hugely entertaining Johnston's rapidly growing popularity is down to his unique interaction with the crowds, as well as the media.

'It's been amazing,' said the 27-year-old. 'It's been such great fun. I guess I'm just a down-to-earth bloke who likes to talk to people. You want people to go home with good memories. I'll chat to anyone from anywhere, as long as they're nice people who are nice to me.'

Watch him on YouTube or Facebook. You'll learn a lot more about the Fire element after a few minutes of looking at him and listening to him talk.

I think he is Outer Fire (Heart Protector/Three Heater), not Inner Fire (Small Intestine/Heart). The difference can often be seen by the way each aspect of Fire talks. Inner Fire, sorting out what it wants to say as it talks, often stumbles or pauses in its attempt to find the right words. Outer Fire is much more smoothly articulate.

◇◇◇◇◇◇◇◇

# 20 JULY 2016
## *Treatment of alopecia – another satisfactory use of a CV/GV block*

Recently, a fellow practitioner, Jo Banthorpe, invited me to her practice for a day in mid-May to help with the treatment of some of her patients. Before I arrived, she warned me that she looked somewhat different from when we had last seen each other because she had developed alopecia, and now had large bare patches on her head. She had therefore shaved her hair close to the skull to make these patches less noticeable. I have Jo's permission to write about this.

During the day with her, I asked her whether she had had treatment for a CV/GV (Ren Mai/DuMai) block, or had even considered this as being the cause of the alopecia. I told her that over the years I had successfully treated several patients with alopecia, each having been told that there was little Western medicine could do to restore hair growth. In each case, clearing a CV/GV block led within a few weeks to the gradual regrowth of the hair. I had been encouraged to select this treatment because I felt that such a drastic depletion of energy causing severe hair loss of this kind could only be the result of some serious energy block. This obviously pointed to a CV/GV block.

I cleared this blockage on Jo during my day with her and awaited the result. You can imagine how happy I was a few days ago to receive an email from her telling me that she was 'Delighted to report that my hair seems to be growing back!' And, 'I don't think it was growing back before we did CV/GV, in fact I think I was still losing it, but more from the hairline at the sides.' She enclosed some photos of the back and side of her head, clearly showing the regrowth of hair.

This is yet another example of the drastic improvement in all kinds of conditions that clearing a CV/GV block can lead to. It isn't always at all clear from our often inadequate pulse readings that there is sufficiently severe depletion of energy to point immediately to a CV/GV block. But if in doubt, and there is a persistent deep-seated condition which your treatment cannot seem to shift, then always think of this block.

I remember quite clearly JR Worsley telling us that if the points for clearing a CV/GV block were on the wrist, we would do it on every patient! Those words have stayed with me for 30 years, and encouraged me to think often of this block and clear it, perhaps receiving confirmation only afterwards, when the patient's symptoms change dramatically, that there was indeed such a block there. So all of you out there who hesitate to diagnose this block because you are uncertain of your pulse-taking or feel reluctant to needle some of these points, just do this treatment. The block is surprisingly often there, and if it isn't, it never hurts to do it. It's only like opening a door which is already open.

◇◇◇◇◇◇◇◇◇

# 25 JULY 2016
## '1 of the 48%'

I am still reeling from the result of the referendum. And I don't agree with many people's passive acceptance that 'Brexit means Brexit'. It certainly doesn't, or at least only if we, who so violently oppose cutting ourselves off from Europe, tamely accept that it does.

So I am on a personal mission to fight what I consider to be the good fight. I have bought some badges supporting the EU, one of which I now wear proudly everywhere. It says '1 of the 48%', and has already provoked an argument from a 'leaver', but also much support from others.

And then I make sure that I buy a copy of the *New European*, which calls itself a 'pop-up newspaper'. It appeared within a week of the referendum, and gives a very healthy European slant to the news. Originally, they said that there were only going to be four weekly copies, as a brief protest against the referendum result, but we're on to copy three now and people are buying it, so I hope it changes its mind and carries on.

I also heard Paddy Ashdown talking on the *Andrew Marr Programme* yesterday morning about a new group he and many others are bringing together called MoreUnited (www.moreunited.uk) which, as he put it so persuasively, is there to give voice to the voiceless, those who don't want to belong to any political party, but feel fervently that Britain should not cut itself off from its international roots. It wants to campaign strongly against the idea that we have to go along with the idea of Brexit, rather than ensuring that we continue to fight against it. So that's another cause I decided to support.

And finally, to my own surprise, as somebody who has always been a floating voter, not attached to any particular party, I have thrown caution to the winds and have joined the Liberal Democrat party, because they are the only party who has said that they will base their plans for the next election solely on fighting to remain in the EU.

So it's been a politically rather hectic few days for me, my pro-European feelings strengthened even more by the terrible events in France and Germany. This is surely not the time to withdraw into an isolationist shell, as though we are trying to tuck ourselves out of sight in this corner of Europe.

◇◇◇◇◇◇◇◇

# 18 AUGUST 2016
## *How to approach treating a patient with breast cancer*

From a five element perspective, the onset of any illness or imbalance of any kind should be interpreted as being the result of some blockage in the balanced flow of life-giving energy round the cycle of the elements. There are many ways in which energy can become blocked, the simplest block being that between mother and child, where for some reason the mother is prevented from passing on enough of her good energy to her child, treated by needling the tonification points. Another form of energy transfer is that between the grandmother and grandchild elements, bypassing the mother element because the grandmother has more energy than the mother to pass on. And then there are all the other forms of blocks, such as Entry/Exit blocks, and the three major blocks, Aggressive Energy, Husband/Wife and Possession.

The important thing when treating somebody who comes to us with a serious condition, as in the case of breast cancer, is not to think that we have to approach treating the patient in any way differently from the way we approach every new patient. We need to go through the same steady first steps of treatment: first trying to diagnose the guardian element, checking for any blocks, beginning with an AE drain, and then concentrating our attention upon strengthening the element we have chosen as much as we can. With a specific diagnosis, such as in the case of breast cancer, we should also think carefully about which particular meridians flow around and through the area of the body where problems are occurring, here the breast, and consider which potential blockages might be occurring there, which have led, may potentially have led or may in the future lead to symptoms appearing. In the case of breast problems, I always needle the points used to clear blocks between Spleen and Heart (a XII/I, Sp/Ht block), and between Kidney and Heart Protector (a IV/V, Ki/HP block). I do this even though my pulse readings may not necessarily indicate these blockages are there, but because needling these points can be regarded as a preventative measure. This will encourage the good flow of energy around the affected breast, and will thus help prevent future blocks occurring. In addition, since pulse interpretation is such a highly skilled art, I never like to rely entirely on my own pulse-reading skills.

If there is already any surgical scarring around this area, the points should only be needled on the healthy, unaffected side, since patients are warned against needling near the scar tissue. Correcting the good flow of energy through a meridian on one side of the body will also help correct its sister flow on the other side.

For further information about how to diagnose and treat blocks, I would refer you to my *Handbook of Five Element Practice* which discusses each block in greater detail.

I have also written two other blogs about Entry/Exit points, one on 14 December 2010 and the other on 22 May 2012, and a blog about treating a patient with terminal cancer on 27 February 2013.

In addition to my blogs, the last chapter of my book *The Pattern of Things* (now published by Singing Dragon under the title of *Patterns of Practice*), entitled *Afterword: Healing in Death*, is my tribute to the courage of a terminally ill cancer patient of mine, and offers a good description of how I approached treating her in the last year of her life.

◇◇◇◇◇◇◇◇◇

# 18 AUGUST 2016
## *Needle retention*

One of the questions I was recently asked on my Facebook Question and Answer sessions was about needle retention. The questioner asked whether there was any difference between manipulating the needle and then leaving it in place, which I interpreted as referring to our five element sedation technique, or removing the needles immediately after needling, our tonification technique. This made me consider carefully what the effect a needle left in the skin has. It is fairly simple to me to understand that when we stimulate a point and remove the needle, we are then handing back to the patient's own energy the task of continuing the effect the tonification needle is intended to produce, without any further interference from the acupuncturist (and I use the word interference advisedly).

But what is actually happening when the needles are left in place, and, as sometimes happens, are stimulated again at intervals? In effect, any needle left in a point continues to activate this point in some way. Sedating a point will therefore draw energy away from the sedated meridian for as long as the needle is inserted. In this case, the acupuncturist continues to treat (to interfere, as I call all treatment) for as long as he/she decides to leave the needle, or more usually the needles, in.

It is interesting that in all the years that I worked under JR's supervision or watched him work with others I cannot remember a single occasion when he said that we should sedate rather than tonify an element, except, of course, for an AE drain and for possession treatment. But for these two treatments the needles are never manipulated whilst in the skin, just repositioned if we feel they are not in the right place or threaten to fall out. I have always interpreted the minimal use of sedation in five element acupuncture as a sign that the initial AE drain on all patients at the first treatment draws away any excess energy from the relevant elements in the patient, leaving us to do what is then needed, which is to stimulate deficient energy, i.e. to tonify and boost the flow of good energy between the elements.

In other forms of acupuncture, it seems that sedation of points by leaving needles in place forms a major role in treatment. I wonder, though, with sedation of this kind which may well calm and pacify energy, what is then done to boost it?

◇◇◇◇◇◇◇◇

## 24 AUGUST 2016
### *Thoughts on the Fire element and other elements prompted by watching Usain Bolt and others at the Rio Olympics*

Usain Bolt is, of course, pure Fire, at the moment the most visible example dominating our headlines. Watching him interact with the crowd has added to my knowledge of Fire, and made me think more of what it tries to offer those around it. So here are some more of my insights.

Fire wants to share its smile, its laughter, its thoughts. If you watch Fire's eyes, they are always looking directly in the eyes of another person when they are talking or smiling or laughing to make sure that their speech, their smiles or their laughter are being received by somebody. You could say that Fire regards them as gifts they want to offer others.

All elements can talk, smile and laugh, but their interactions will be directed outwards in different ways because they come from a different space within them, created, as everything we do is, by a particular guardian element. Wood wants to command attention, point something out. Earth wants to ensure that all within hearing respond to it, for it likes being at the centre of a circle, not demanding one-to-one attention. Metal, true to its natural desire to observe and judge life from a distance, will tend to keep many things to itself, saying the minimum that it thinks needs to be said, often choosing to keep its thoughts to itself, unless actively asked to share them. Its smiles and its laughter are more like brief flashes breaking out, as though disturbing its preference for silence. Compare, for example, the quiet celebration of joy that Jessica Ennis (Metal, I think) shows at winning with Usain Bolt's tumultuous one, where he draws the whole world around him, spectators and TV audiences alike, to help him share his joy.

Finally, there is Water, always last in my list, because it is such a mysterious element and so difficult for me to pin down, with its often rather hysterical outpourings of speech and emotion, which are more likely to make us step away rather than draw us towards it, because it makes us feel unsure of what we are experiencing and how we should be reacting.

I use a study of myself, as Fire, more than of anybody else in trying to fathom the secrets of what Fire wants of life. Thinking of Usain Bolt, as I was this morning, I realized that my need to share my thoughts appears in the urge behind my teaching and my writing, particularly of my blogs. And I want to share my thoughts immediately, almost unable to wait until I have somebody with me, either in person or through social media of some kind, with whom to share them. I can't not share, just as Usain Bolt can't not smile.

A comment from India from a very perceptive Water patient of mine after she read this blog:

I just wanted say how nice it was to read your blog about the elements today. Of course the one on Water is very apt, based on my own experience. I think Water surges out towards people it feels comfortable with (or communicative towards) but maybe tends to overdo it, leaving a confused or uncomfortable gap.

◇◇◇◇◇◇◇◇

## 26 AUGUST 2016
### *The challenge of treating very young children*

In the early days of my practice I was very reluctant to treat young children. I knew that they could not themselves tell me what was wrong, and without talking to them I was not sure how I was going to diagnose their element. Everything I learnt about them would therefore have to be filtered through what their parent told me. (For simplicity's sake, I will call the mother the parent, although the same holds true for the father.) Before seeing the child, therefore, we need to arrange to talk to the mother quietly on her own, and not in the child's hearing. Ideally, this should be done face to face, rather than on the phone, and certainly not by email. A private talk will also yield crucial information about the mother's relationship to the child, and here we have to use our diagnostic skills to discover what exactly is going on between mother and child.

Most, if not all, problems in young children (and in later life!) originate in family life. The difficulty for us here is that most parents are often unaware of the part they play in this, for, like most of us when faced with unpleasant facts, we are reluctant to admit to our own responsibility. A parent of a distressed child often has unresolved issues around being a parent, which may well be, and usually is, the prime reason for disturbance in the child. I have some very good examples of this from my own practice which have reinforced my conviction that if only I could treat the mother, the young child would probably not need treatment. This conviction, and often my experiences of failing to help the child, have reinforced my increasing reluctance over the years to treat young children.

I was fortunate that I was able to take the first two children I was asked to treat to see JR Worsley. This was at a very early stage in my practice, when I did not know how I should approach treating them. The first child was a young boy of about three, who was said by his mother to be completely out of control. He would only let his mother touch him, refused to relate to anybody else and had been given a provisional diagnosis of autism. His mother and I had to drag him kicking and screaming from the car to the practice room, where JR, after looking at him quickly, told me to carry out the AE drain, despite his loud protests, with his mother and me holding him firmly on my lap. As I recall, there was no AE, although I have since often found a surprising amount of AE in even the youngest child.

JR diagnosed the element as Wood, and told me to follow the AE drain with the source points on Wood on the left side only. To my surprise, shortly after the treatment, the young boy suddenly fell quiet, turned his head to look at me and kept eye contact as I walked away, something he had not done with any of us before. I interpreted this as the Wood element diffusing his terrible sense of anger. From then on, for the few treatments he continued to come to me once a fortnight for the simple five element command point treatment JR had recommended, he would run happily to greet me as though he enjoyed his treatments. Nobody would then have diagnosed him as other than a normal little boy.

Sadly, however, I was only allowed to treat him a few more times. JR had pointed out that I should do possession treatment on the mother, luckily a patient of mine, something I had not yet noted, but very shortly afterwards, the mother abruptly stopped treatment for both herself and her child. The child's father, who was very happy with my continuing to treat his son, explained his wife's decision to stop treatment by the fact that she was very disturbed to think that I might think that she was the cause of the child's problems, something she denied totally. He himself could see that she was much too possessive of the child, but could do little to persuade her to allow me to continue treating their child.

I had similar experiences with two other mothers, both of whom, though ostensibly wanting help for their young children, refused to acknowledge that there was anything in their own attitudes to their children which might be contributing to the problem, and both quickly discontinued the child's treatment very early on despite quite clear evidence that it was helping.

Of course, other practitioners may have had happier experiences of treating children than I have had, and their experiences may well be with less complex mother–child relationships than mine have been. I'm sure, too, that much can be done to help young children deal with whatever problems, psychological or physical, they come to you with simply by trying hard to diagnose the element by means of any information you can glean, then doing an AE drain and basic five element treatment.

I am happy, though, that I can finish this blog with a rather lovely story of the successful treatment of a young child, though I never saw the child or inserted a single needle. A patient of mine had an 18-month-old daughter who had suddenly started to suffer from asthma. Could I do something to help, she asked me. With some of the unhappy experiences I had had in mind, I was at first reluctant to do so, but then I put on my five element hat, and asked myself, 'Why would a little baby develop asthma? Why would its Metal element be in such distress?' Metal, being the element of our relationship to our father, I asked whether anything had recently changed at home, particularly in relation to the child's father. She told me that he had joined a golf club, and was now away from home for much of the weekend. Before this, the whole family had had happy weekends doing things together. I talked through the needs of the Metal element with both father and mother, and suggested that the father should make every effort to be with the child as much as he could, perhaps sacrificing some golf for his child's sake. This was rather a long shot on my behalf, and I wasn't very optimistic that this would help.

To the father's credit, he did this, and even I was surprised when the mother told me that, after a few weeks of increased attention from the father, the child's asthma started to improve, and eventually disappeared altogether. And this without the need for any medication, or any needles. Here, both parents had enough insight into family relationships and were open to listening to advice, something which is unfortunately rather rare, as we know.

∞∞∞∞∞∞

# 12 SEPTEMBER 2016
## *We comfort eat when we don't get enough comfort from eating*

A few days ago I was sitting in my favourite café enjoying my favourite meal of the day, which is breakfast – a small espresso with a drop of very hot milk and a fresh croissant to dunk into it. I was contemplating the world around me, thinking how good it was peacefully to savour the taste of what I was eating, when a thought popped into my mind, which was how important it is to give ourselves the time to enjoy food.

That led me to think how little attention we often now pay to the simple pleasure of eating when we can dash into a coffee house and grab a quick drink and a bite to eat on our way to hurrying to wherever we are going. This made me consider what this is doing to our Earth element, our mother element which is there to nourish and support the other elements, and which needs to be nourished and supported itself if it is to do its work properly. It has to learn how to do this, as all elements do, as they gradually take over the role their mother has taken on in the womb. I now watch with dismay as mothers stuff bottles into small babies' mouths in their prams in the street or even in buses amidst all the tumult and traffic noise. Here there is none of the peaceful enjoyment of feeding time which we should be allowing our babies, and which help its tender little Earth element to assume its role.

I wonder how far our lack of attention to the actual process of enjoying the food we put in our mouths, particularly in the early days of a child's life, is one of the reasons for the sharp rise in obesity we see all around us. The Earth element can only develop as it should in a loving, caring environment, where it is able to welcome food as something which warms and nourishes it. It needs this to sustain a healthy relationship to food throughout later life. If it is denied this comfort because its Stomach official is asked to snatch at the food that reaches it, it will try to hold on to as much of this food as it can, being unwilling to discard what is unwanted because it is not given enough time to process it. Rather than satisfying it, then, the food that reaches it is tantalizingly snatched away as it is gobbled down in the hurly-burly of modern life.

This may perhaps be one of the reasons behind the success of so many TV cookery programmes. Do we, through them at one remove as it were, learn to enjoy again, or even for the first time, the delights of food cooked as it should be, as though we are kidding ourselves that this is how we are feeding ourselves? Is this, too, the reason for the runaway success of *The Great British Bake Off*, with a mother or a grandmother substitute for the whole country so clearly there in Mary Berry, as the TV immerses us in succulent images of home-baked cakes, so Earth-like a delight?

Somewhere hidden in this, too, may well lie the reason why I hardly pass a person in the street who is not holding a cup of coffee or tea in their hands, often making no attempt to drink it, a substitute for a mother's nipple if there ever was one, as though their Earth element is sending out a constant reminder to them of its need for attention.

And is this, too, why I so enjoy sitting in a coffee house with my coffee and croissant, a reminder, perhaps, of home and hearth (and mother) all those years ago?

◇◇◇◇◇◇◇◇

# 4 OCTOBER 2016
## *For simplicity's sake – another heartfelt plea*

Anybody who knows anything about me will know how often I plead for one basic principle of five element acupuncture, which is to keep it simple. I always hear JR Worsley's voice in my ear telling us that we really only need three minutes with our patients: one to look at them, one to decide on the point(s) to needle and one to say goodbye. It was said jokingly (or at least I assumed it was), but, like everything he said, it hides profound wisdom. The longer I practise, the more I have come to understand this.

As all good five element acupuncturists know, the aim of treatment is to hand control back to the elements within the patient as quickly as possible. All treatment represents an interference with a patient's natural energy, a temporary taking-over of control. We were always told that it is not we who heal our patients; it is nature which does this through the elements which create the world outside and create our bodies and within them our souls. So if we can find out where a hitch has occurred in the beautiful, health-giving flow of energy round the cycle of the elements, and help reinstate this natural flow, our work is done and we should withdraw from the scene.

From this viewpoint, it can then be regarded as a waste of energy to spend so much time mulling over the actions of individual points rather than trying to pinpoint the element under stress and choosing points relating to that element. Sadly, though, I see too many people doing this. We can call this 'not seeing the wood for the trees'.

There is no doubt that it requires much humility to accept that observing the work of the elements in a human being demands skills which we can only acquire over time and involves much hard work. For example, I like to tell people that it took me many years accurately to recognize the fear at the heart of the Water element, or that flushed red cheeks did not, as I assumed, point to Fire, but either to Wood or Earth out of control. (In the case of Wood, it is because it is depriving its child Fire of the warmth it needs, and therefore Fire tries to stoke it up artificially; or, in the case of Earth, it is because its mother, Fire, is out of control and passes on too much Fire to its child. Fire never has permanently flushed skin. Its colour flushes and then fades again quite quickly. It often has a kind of blotchy red look.) It took me a long time and much evidence from treating patients to recognize this and to accept that this was so.

But once we realize that what we need to do is study people as closely as possible wherever we encounter them (TV or cafés are good places to observe the significant interactions which point to one element or another), and gradually to build up a personal filing system of indicators for each element, then practice becomes simpler and simpler. The mantra, as always, is: 'Find the element and the points look after themselves'. I don't think it matters at all if I choose one point and another practitioner chooses another, provided both strengthen the patient's guardian element.

◇◇◇◇◇◇◇◇

# 12 OCTOBER 2016
## *Off on my tenth visit to China*

I will be getting on the plane to Beijing tomorrow where Mei, Guy and I will be giving two seminars. The first will be over five days, for about 120 students, nearly all of whom we have not seen before. To attend this seminar, they must first have taken part in one of the introductory five element courses given by former students of ours, a healthy sign of how many acupuncturists over there already feel competent enough to teach others. The second two-day seminar is for a more advanced group of about 50 practitioners, all of whom have come to some of our previous seminars.

Finally, to round off our visit on our last day, something quite different is planned. The day will be spent at the Institute of Acupuncture of the China Academy of Chinese Medical Science, a Chinese medicine research institute under the State Administration of Traditional Chinese Medicine. I am told that it is responsible for 17 research institutes, six medical organizations, two pharmaceutical companies and a publishing house. It has been working with the World Health Organization and has established three centres of clinical research into acupuncture and traditional Chinese medicine. In the morning the Institute will be host to the inaugural meeting of the new Five Element Acupuncture Association. This is an umbrella association covering those teaching five element acupuncture according to the principles handed on to them during the seminars we have held over the past five years. As we know, there is always a risk that some may set themselves up as experts in their field based upon little practical experience, and this is particularly true of acupuncture in China where many thousands of practitioners now qualify from universities of traditional Chinese medicine each year. The association will be aimed at ensuring that those intending to teach this particular branch of five element acupuncture are qualified to do so. In the afternoon we will be holding a seminar for the Institute of Acupuncture, making this a very full last day indeed.

As usual, I am taking quite a few books with me as presents, including children's books for some of the babies born to graduates of our previous seminars, some more of my books as presentation copies to the various institutes, and, this time, a selection of Monkey Press books which Sandra Hill has kindly donated, and which they are not familiar with over there. I am also taking a selection of my own books which my publisher, Singing Dragon, has asked me to pass on to the Chinese publisher who has now signed an agreement with them for the publication of translations of my other four books, in addition to the translation of my *Handbook of Five Element Practice* (the book, which I proudly tell everybody, has already sold more than 20,000 copies over there). Mei has already translated my *Simple Guide*, and it is in the process of being published. Translations of the other three books, the *Keepers of the Soul* (my very favourite book), *Patterns of*

*Practice* and *On Being a Five Element Acupuncturist* (my blog book, I call it), are also already in the pipeline.

So a lot of things are happening in China on the five element acupuncture front, something I feel I am blessed to witness and to participate in.

I will report back further on my return to London at the end of October.

◇◇◇◇◇◇◇◇

# 27 OCTOBER 2016
## *Thoughts on my return from China*

So here I am sitting comfortably once again in my favourite London coffee shop, and feeling as though the past ten days in China have been like a dream and never happened. This is always how I feel on my return from such a different environment and culture. I am suffering a bit from jet-lag after our 11-hour flight, but not as much as I normally do, because Guy has given me a tip on how to combat jet-lag. This is for acupuncturists only, I'm afraid, but consists in needling the horary points of the elements whose times we are entering as we move from one time-zone to another. It does seem to work, although not every time, I found. Certainly, after self-needling a series of points during sleepless intervals during the night, I woke this morning experiencing none of the heavy jet-lag I normally feel.

On our flight back, Guy and I enjoyed ourselves mulling over the very happy days we had spent with our students on the two seminars we held, and making plans for what we will be doing at our next scheduled visit in April 2017. We always say that the seminar we have just completed is our best, but these two truly were the best, because we saw such an improvement in five element practice even in the short time since we were last in China. I often feel that the enthusiasm and dedication our Chinese students show put our Western-based students to shame. It is such a joy for me to see how what started in 2011 with a mere 15 students in Nanning has now grown five years later to many hundreds of practitioners throughout China. This is an awesome achievement, and makes me very proud of all the work everybody has put into developing five element acupuncture there – from Professor Liu Lihong who first invited me, through Mei and Guy, and on to every one of those who have moved the study of five element acupuncture forward to where it is at present in China.

I would like to dedicate this blog to all who made our latest visit such a rewarding one, and in particular Lynn Yang who organized everything so beautifully, as she always does, and held everything together, from the moment of our arrival at Beijing Airport to that of our departure. I would also like to thank her and Caroline who acted as such splendid translators for us. And then we owe a great deal of the success of our visit to a small army of helpers who took much of the strain of organizing the very large group of well over 100 acupuncturists into orderly ranks so that they could observe treatments in the practice rooms in small batches. All of these helpers together made my tenth visit to China such a successful and joyous event.

# 11 NOVEMBER 2016
## *A new world order perhaps?*

I find it exhilarating – both fascinating and appalling – to be a witness to the enormous events of the past few months, now culminating in Trump's triumph. These events are called seismic, because, like earthquakes, they burst out and demolished much of the old political order. First we had Brexit, and now we have Trump (Brexit, Brexit plus plus as he himself said). Brexit was bad enough to deal with, and many of us, me included, are still unable properly to deal with it (which is why I now wear a badge proudly proclaiming 'Brexit does not mean Brexit', to be obtained from Joy Gerrard at www.visibleanger.com, who very kindly designed this at my request).

Being appalled by what is happening in this country and the US is, in my view, easy, but to see this as forming part of some kind of important trend in the history of the world is much harder to envisage. This only became possible for me after I heard Madeleine Albright, the US Senator and former Secretary of State, giving a very illuminating talk on the BBC *Today* programme yesterday. Among other things, she said that 'the social contract has been broken. People are talking to their government with 21st-century technology, the government hears them with 20th-century technology, and answers them with 19th-century technology.' I interpret this as meaning that there is a huge disconnect between how we are now governed and how we need to be governed in this new world of ours. And what can be seen as the protest votes of all those who supported Jeremy Corbyn or voted for Brexit or have sent Trump to the White House are all signs of this huge disconnect.

Perhaps we are now seeing the last dying struggles of the old order, in which the money and power of the elite 1 percent has dominated over the feelings of inadequacy and abandonment of the remaining 99 per cent. Seen from this viewpoint, the triumphs of Jeremy Corbyn, the Brexiteers and Trump represent a powerful uprising of those who feel dispossessed and marginalized against an established order which has so far always favoured the advantaged, a sad symbol of this being the mantra of 'austerity' imposed for many years upon the disadvantaged in many countries from Greece to this country.

Maybe, then, what we are seeing happening now is the death throes of one world order and the inevitable birth pangs of another hopefully more enlightened one. It may be fanciful of me to hope that this is so, but hope is what we need when what has seemed to be a dark pall of despair has hung over us for so long. We need now to hope for a breakthrough to a better world which will build itself slowly on the ruins of the breakdown we are witnessing today.

This is why I like to read the blog written by Yanis Varoufakis, the former Greek Finance Minister, to be found at https://yanisvaroufakis.eu, because he and those working with him throughout the world are endeavouring to make the case for a new world order. This gives me hope that there are enough people out there not content just to complain about the state of the world but to do something about it.

◇◇◇◇◇◇◇◇

# 17 NOVEMBER 2016
## *The filter our element lays between us and the world*

The more I try to teach people about the elements, the more I realize that over the years I have worked out my own personal, possibly rather idiosyncratic way of interpreting the signals a patient's elements are sending me, and using these as pointers to a particular element. I imagine that all experienced five element acupuncturists must do the same. None of these pointers will be exactly those that other practitioners have discovered, because everything we experience has to pass through the filter with which our guardian element envelops us. Some of the impressions we receive from a patient may have some similarity with those which others will experience, but we will each put our own interpretation upon them.

I was reminded of this a few days ago when I ran a seminar with Guy Caplan. He is Metal and I am Fire, so inevitably we see life through two very different filters. This was emphasized for me when both of us were interacting with a very lively Fire patient. As usual, whenever I am in the presence of Fire in another person, I relax because I can feel that I am on familiar ground. So this particular patient, though very much out-of-control Fire, did not prove a problem for me to deal with. On the contrary, I felt I knew exactly how she needed to be treated, which was in a robust, quite challenging way, my Fire, as it were, blazing away to control her overheated Fire. Guy, on the other hand, told me that he found her exaggerated gaiety uncomfortable to deal with, and would have taken longer to work out how to react to it and contain it. We can interpret this as hot Fire threatening to melt Metal, whilst hot Fire just makes me feel not perhaps always completely comfortable to be with, but certainly not difficult to deal with.

This is why as practitioners we should do all that we can to find out what our particular element is, recognize its qualities, make allowances for its weaknesses and take all these factors into account when dealing with our patients. This is not an easy task, because we all have a tendency to think that when we have an uneasy relationship with our patient the fault lies in them not in us. It is good to remind ourselves at intervals that this is not so. Often it is the balance of the elements within us, particularly that of our guardian element, that is shaping our relationship to our patient, and perhaps distorting it in some way which we fail to recognize.

◇◇◇◇◇◇◇◇◇

# 23 NOVEMBER 2016
## *Words, words, words!*

So many words to read in so many different books and in so many different languages, and so little time to do this in! I have a large pile of books sitting waiting for me to read – books I have borrowed from the local library (most of them), books I have bought secondhand from Oxfam or online, and then (just a few) books I have bought for myself using a generous book token given to me for my birthday a few weeks ago.

Looking at this pile, I realize again, as I have increasingly begun to realize, that I have no chance of rereading any but a few of the many of my own books filling my bookcases. Sometimes I look longingly at volumes of Marcel Proust (in French, of course – being a linguist), which are waiting hopefully for me to open their pages again, many, many years after I used them to work on as part of an (unsuccessful) postgraduate degree. I say to myself that if I decide to submerge myself once again in Proust's glorious French, I will not be able to read anything new for at least a few months – and I don't want to sacrifice for this the time I would like to dedicate to discovering some exciting new writer who will open my eyes to a new world of words.

The only writers I have regularly reread in the past are some of the classical authors, such as Dickens, Trollope or George Eliot, and, perhaps considered slightly odd, some old-fashioned detective stories which belonged to my mother and to which I return again and again as they envelop me in a familiar and comfortable world of the past, such as Ellis Peters or Patricia Wentworth.

I am now an absolute font of knowledge about good detective stories. As for many people, they are my escape into a fantasy world where the good always triumphs and the bad is eventually defeated. In the real world, the opposite often seems to be true, and particularly so now. In these very uncertain times, I need an escape route like this which goes some way to relieving some of the distress I feel at what is happening in the world outside.

◇◇◇◇◇◇◇◇

# 5 DECEMBER 2016
## *The pitfalls of making snap diagnoses*

Since all five element acupuncturists know that diagnosing a patient's element takes much time and is certainly not done in an instant, it is obvious that trying to do the same by looking at the necessarily brief glimpses of politicians and other famous people on television or social media can at best be a rather hit-and-miss affair, and at worst may lead us to making completely erroneous conclusions. I remember well that I was convinced that Julia Roberts was Fire, because this is how I interpreted her endless smiling. I told all my students this until one day, a good few years later, when my understanding of the different qualities of the elements had obviously deepened, I noticed a different reaction in me to this smile. It certainly did not warm me, but, instead, irritated me with what I now thought was its artificiality. I realized suddenly that, rather than giving me something, as Fire always tries to do, it was demanding something of me. Once I had noticed this, I changed my diagnosis from Fire to Earth, and have stuck with that ever since. This was a good warning to me always to hedge my conclusions about elements with a few question marks.

So, now being an older and wiser observer of my fellow human beings, I hesitate a bit in offering my thoughts on the elements of politicians much in the news at the moment, but if I don't add my slice of knowledge to what others are trying to learn about the elements, then I think that is a bit cowardly. Those of us who have been looking at the elements for many years (in my case over 35 years) have a duty to pass on whatever they have learnt to those with less experience. So here goes with what I have observed in two politicians very much in the news at the moment: Theresa May, in this country, and Donald Trump, in the United States.

At such a difficult time for the world, I find it interesting and disturbing that the fate of so many people is in the hands of two people I consider to be of the Wood element. Leaving aside their politics, what is it about the Wood element which makes me wary of this element being the guiding force in a leader of a country (and in Trump's case in a leader of the Western world)? I've thought carefully about this, and will continue to do so as I observe their words and their actions over the next crucial months. Here I can draw on the knowledge of the Wood element I have gained through my acupuncture practice. If we think of the cycle of the elements as describing the arc of a human life from birth to death, then after its period of gestation in the seed of all life, the Water element, life emerges into the open in the Wood element, at its point of birth, and then on to early childhood. I ask myself whether I want my leaders to express the childlike qualities which the Wood element can often show.

What, then, are Wood's qualities which will manifest themselves in the positions of power held by a country's leaders? It definitely has a lot of strength and stamina, good qualities in a leader. Its principal emotion is a kind of forcefulness of character which demands that others do what it wants them to do, but can express itself in outbursts of anger if others around it do not fall in with its plans. We see this kind of anger very clearly in Donald Trump's emotional outbursts and also the lack of control which accompanies them. Wood does not yet have the maturity to rein in this anger if this would be a wiser course to take. Theresa May, too, though much less overtly Wood-like than Donald Trump, shows flashes of anger if a situation does not please her. A constituent of hers at a meeting with her said that she became very irritated when questioned too closely. Observing her on a BBC programme, I noticed that as the camera panned back to her after I suspect she thought she was no longer on public view, she looked surprisingly cross – not at all the bland, controlled persona she had shown us during the interview itself.

So it will be very interesting to see how these two leaders deal with the inevitably difficult times which lie ahead for them. It does not therefore surprise me that, as of this date, 5 December, Theresa May has not yet come up with any clear plans for how to proceed with Brexit. Though planning and decision making are the prerogative of the Wood element, they can easily lead, on the one hand, to over-dogmatic statements ('Brexit means Brexit' being one of them), and, on the other, to hesitancy, if the Wood element is under stress. And who, in the positions of power which May and Trump hold, will not be under stress in one form or other? Rather worryingly for both of them, this sense of balance in their Wood element seems rather to be absent, in Trump's case most obviously so, his Tweets being clear evidence of this. Theresa May, too, certainly made some hasty, rather odd decisions soon after coming to power (reinstatement of grammar schools and delaying a decision on the Hinkley Point nuclear power station). One of these decisions (grammar schools) has since disappeared without trace, and she rescinded the other very quickly and rather ignominiously in the light of China's anger.

She has said that thinking about what to do about Brexit keeps her awake at night. Rather amusingly, I see this as a clear sign of the struggles her Wood element is undergoing to keep everything on track as it passes through its horary time between 11 pm at night and 3 am in the morning. Angry as I am about all the unnecessary expenditure which will be spent on the Brexit negotiations and would much better be spent on care homes for the elderly or children's playgrounds for the young, I know I will still find it fascinating to observe how what I consider to be these two clear examples of the Wood element in power will deal with that power.

◇◇◇◇◇◇◇◇

# 7 DECEMBER 2016
## *How the elements cope with responsibility*

Having written about the Wood element in positions of power in my last blog (posted 5 December), I feel I should turn my attention to the other elements. Most obvious of all is a very clear representative of the Metal element, Barack Obama (with, standing at his shoulder, one of the greatest statesmen of them all, Nelson Mandela). I can think of no greater antithesis to Donald Trump than Obama. Where Trump is impulsive, given to displays of uncoordinated thought and action, we have in Obama the very epitome of the opposite, somebody who thinks things through carefully, utters no unconsidered word or action, stands back, observes and only then acts or speaks. Trump's impulsive tweeting would be anathema to Metal.

So I am left to consider the remaining three elements, Fire, Earth and Water. As those who have read my *Keepers of the Soul* (Chapter 6) already know, over the years I have always used Tony Blair as an excellent example of one aspect of the Fire element, Inner Fire (Small Intestine). This side of Fire has a toughness coming from its need to sort things appropriately for the Heart, and will feel that it must refuse to do what it does not consider right to do, and force through what it thinks right. Whatever our opinion of Tony Blair's decision about the Iraq war, he was convinced, and is still convinced, that this was necessary, and would not allow public opinion, so vehemently against him at the time, to sway him. There was, too, the added pressure exerted upon him from his association with George Bush (another Wood leader to go with Donald Trump and Theresa May), who drew Tony Blair in his wake.

I think that the other side of Fire, Outer Fire, is well represented by two flamboyant politicians, Boris Johnson and Nigel Farage, both able to attract supporters by acting the clown and making them laugh, a very different Fire quality to that of Tony Blair.

Fire and Wood are the two strong yang, outward-facing elements keen to push themselves forward. We can contrast that here with Obama's Metal, with its inward-turning yin qualities.

We are now left with the last two elements, Earth and Water. Interestingly, what I consider to be the most powerful element of all, Water, does not like to push itself too strongly into the limelight, as befits its deeply yin nature, making it the most hidden of all elements, as it works away in the dark. The most obvious politician I can think of to show Water's characteristics is Gordon Brown, briefly a Prime Minister, and yet somebody who for many years attempted to undermine Tony Blair and usurp his position. When faced with the first opportunity to challenge Blair, though, he hesitated and retreated, only becoming Prime Minister once Tony Blair had resigned. And as Prime Minister, despite so desperately wanting this position for so many years, he was surprisingly hesitant and uneasy in the limelight.

Finally, Earth, for which, David Cameron, our former Prime Minister, is a good example. Here is a man at ease with himself, and easy in the company of others, with one of those soothing Earth voices. Once having made the fatal decision to hold the referendum, he was unable to deal with its consequences, resigning immediately rather than facing them. Powerful when surrounded by others in power (the yang aspect of Earth), Earth's yielding yin aspect came to the fore when he lost the referendum, and like Gordon Brown, but for other reasons, he retreated rapidly into the background. In the last glimpse of him on the Downing Street doorstep, he was, appropriately for Earth, closely surrounded by his family.

Some people reading these thoughts of mine will disagree with my conclusions, but I hope what I have written has at least made them think a little more about how the elements, in shaping all of us, shape our politicians in very specific ways. These may often be disturbing ways, but equally often, I hope, positive ones, too. After all, South Africa would still be under the thrall of apartheid if there had been no Nelson Mandela. I hold fast to my thoughts of him as a good antidote to fearing what Trump may unleash upon the world.

◇◇◇◇◇◇◇◇

# 11 DECEMBER 2016
## *An attempt to demystify the term 'possession' in five element acupuncture*

There is much discussion going on at the moment in China around the use of the term in five element acupuncture which in English we call 'possession'. I gather that the Mandarin word that has been used to translate it has all the overtones which the English word has. I have always felt that this is an unfortunate term, but one that is so embedded in five element practice that I have been reluctant to discard it and seek another, less charged one. But now, because of the Chinese hesitancy in continuing to use it, it seems the right time to think again whether we need to change it to make it describe more accurately and appropriately the condition patients suffer from.

I need first to define my understanding of the condition itself before trying to come up with a suitable new term for it. It will help by describing what is, in effect, the very simple test we use to diagnose it. Here the practitioner looks very closely straight into one of the patient's eyes, and assesses how the patient reacts to this strongly focused look. In everyday life, it is rare for us to stare straight into somebody's eyes in this way, unless in an aggressive or very loving way. In the normal course of events, such an intense stare becomes uncomfortable both for the person staring and for the person being stared it, so that both will try to break off this close eye contact as soon as possible. As a diagnostic tool in five element acupuncture, we are looking to see whether the patient does not react as expected, but instead continues to maintain eye contact without any apparent sign of discomfort. In a non-possessed patient, there will be an almost immediate movement to the eye, a blink or a turning away, as evidence of the natural discomfort felt at being stared at in this way. In possessed people, however, this does not happen; the patient continues to stare unblinkingly at the practitioner.

This is the only, I repeat only, fail-safe way to diagnose this condition. If present, it then requires a specific treatment which will clear it if done properly. For the actual procedure, I would refer you to my *Handbook of Five Element Practice* (Chapter 7 in the new Singing Dragon edition), which describes this in detail.

I have thought a great deal about what can cause possession, and then why the term seems to me to be an inaccurate and therefore misleading description, however ingrained it is in five element practice. Most of my learning has come from observing my patients, chief amongst which is my experience of treating a young woman many years ago. She had come for help to enable her to overcome her inability to sit down and eat with other people, having instead always to eat on her own. She could not tell me when this fear of eating with others had started, nor could she think of any particular reason to explain it. A few minutes after I had carried out the possession treatment, she said suddenly, 'When my mother went blind when I was six…' When I expressed my amazement that she had not told me this before, she was surprised to learn that she had not, adding, 'They took me away to stay with my grandmother, and I thought my mother had died. That was when I started to refuse to eat with other people.' I realized then that the treatment had unlocked a door to her past which had been closed since her childhood. I have had similar experiences with other patients, where the possession treatment opened up some past history which was hindering them from living a full life.

I have come to regard possession as a form of defence mechanism protecting a patient from reliving some overpowering previous experience, a way of shutting themselves off from continuing to experience something that originally overwhelmed them. When I was studying many years ago, one of my tutors told us that he regarded possession simply as a more extreme form of obsession, a condition in which the patient tries to gain some control over something which has overwhelmed them, whilst, in most cases, still managing to lead an apparently normal life. In some people, however, such experiences become so overpowering that they cannot be controlled and can lead to serious psychological conditions, such as schizophrenia.

I do not regard possession as being the result of the invasion of some external force which the term might seem to imply. I see it instead as an internal mechanism that patients develop to help them cope with a very difficult situation which they cannot deal with in any other way. It is as though they put up a protective glass screen behind which they can hide themselves from the world, but which is often not visible to those around them. My young patient had been living an apparently normal life, except with regard to her eating arrangements. Possession should always therefore be seen as an escape route taken by those subject to some intolerable inner pain.

It is not easy to think of a good replacement term which removes the connection to other uses of the term that have a religious or mystical bias. I am thinking this through carefully, and the only alternative I can think of at the moment is the term 'Internal Dragons'. This is the name given to one of the group of seven acupuncture points used in this treatment. I remember being told some years ago that the seven points we use could be regarded as seven dragons chasing away seven demons, an image I liked. This may again come a little too close to the concept of possession as occurring as a result of some invasion from outside, a kind of take-over by an alien force. However, we can think of demons in much the same way as we talk of a person being subject to the 'demon drink', something somebody brings upon themselves, not something which attacks them from outside.

It is heart-warming to me that five element acupuncture has such a simple and profound treatment protocol for helping restore to good health people suffering from such dislocation in their lives, and one which can break down the internal barrier that life has forced them to place between themselves and the world outside. I find the image of calling upon kindly dragons to fight the internal demons which are trying to take control of our patients' lives strangely comforting.

If I, and others around me, can find a better term which satisfies the Chinese objections, I will pass this on in a future blog.

# 2017 BLOGS

◇◇◇◇◇◇◇◇

# 4 JANUARY 2017
## *Measuring life with coffee spoons*

It is with delight that I come across pieces of writing which make me laugh because of their rightness. I came across two such this week, one after the other in the space of a few hours, and here they are.

I heard the first during a day's reading of TS Eliot poems on the BBC. One of his lines reads:

I have measured out my life with coffee spoons.

The second was something I heard the art critic John Berger saying, when he was talking about writing, and which formed part of the TV obituary on his death a few days ago:

[Writing] helps me make sense of things.

Both sayings resonate deeply with me. As people who know me will recognize, I, too, appear to measure out my life with the coffee spoons I use to stir the many espressos I like to drink in the many different coffee houses around London in which I do my thinking and my writing.

And writing, which is something I have found I have to do, does indeed 'help me make sense of things'. My writing helps me make sense not only of my work as an acupuncturist, but of my life in general. So it is with great joy that I welcome these two quotations into my collection of sayings that enrich my life.

◇◇◇◇◇◇◇◇◇

# 20 JANUARY 2017
## *Being incurably curious*

I have just passed a lovely sign on the outside of the Wellcome Collection in the Marylebone Road here in London. Appropriately for its name and for what it does, which is focused on medicine and helping the ill, it says in bold letters: 'Welcome to the Incurably Curious.' On the bus ride back home, I decided that it would be good to adopt this as my own catchphrase, but with a slight modification. This would amend it slightly to read 'Welcome to the Curably Curious', in honour of my calling as an acupuncturist, because it is our curiosity, in five element terms, which, far from 'killing the cat' as the saying goes, helps us to cure.

And curiosity is what we need – an infinite dose of it throughout every minute of our working lives to help us understand our patients better and through this understanding restore them to good health.

I have always been incurably curious, from childhood onwards, staring unashamedly at people to try to fathom what makes them tick, and how they relate to others. I think people have always at some level puzzled me, challenging my Small Intestine to understand what is going on in another person at every new encounter. I suppose it was therefore only natural that I would eventually gravitate towards a calling which feeds my desire to explore the intricacies of human relationships, however late in my life this was, for I only started practising acupuncture in my mid-40s, exactly at the midpoint of my life when viewed from my present standpoint. I am a living example of the dictum that it is never too late to change the direction of one's life, and that it is often only by passing through the dark days that light begins to shine through.

For I came across acupuncture – or, as I like to think somewhat fancifully, acupuncture found me – at a crossroads in my life, with the early part of my adult life, that of being wife and mother, almost behind me, and the next part hidden behind what seemed to me to be an impenetrable fog. So the moment I encountered acupuncture for the first time surprised me with its rightness; it opened a door wide on to a completely new vision of life which has fascinated me, occupied me and preoccupied me ever since.

As a coda to this blog, I have just read the following passage in a book by Barney Norris called *Five Rivers Meet on a Wooded Plain* (a lovely title in itself). This seems to me to describe very acutely what intrigues me so much about encountering other people:

> So I love watching the way another person holds themselves when they are alone and thinking. Their actions and postures are windows into the vast and secret worlds below the surface of the day around me, the lives of others.

I love the thought of those 'vast and secret worlds' which surround me.

◇◇◇◇◇◇◇◇◇

# 8 FEBRUARY 2017
## *The taking of 'selfies'*

The following is a quotation from a book I am reading at the moment. It is a detective story, and its author has many interesting insights into life. The book is called *Death in the*

*Tuscan Hills* by Marco Vichi. Here he is describing somebody who is leafing through a photo album.

> He retired to the kitchen with a box of old family photos... Photos were ruthless. They showed moments lost for ever, people long since dead. They were an attempt to cheat death, a painful illusion, and looking at them made one more aware than ever that time was a mystery.
>
> After looking at them all one by one, he closed the box of memories with a sigh.

Perhaps, indeed, people's recent mania for the constant taking of photos, usually of themselves, rather than giving themselves time to observe life at first hand through their own eyes, is part of an attempt to 'cheat death', to reassure ourselves that we are alive. I observe with some incredulity and much sadness this endless taking of photos, the living of life at one remove which this represents. So many pieces of electronic equipment, such as smartphones with their numerous gadgets, now put a barrier up between people and the world around them. I wonder what effect this is having on our personal relationships.

I was also saddened recently to hear that, far from connecting people to one another, as Facebook is intended to do, it can have just the opposite effect, that of isolating people. I have been told that young girls can now spend hours alone in their rooms taking photo upon photo of themselves until they are satisfied with the one they eventually feel is good enough to send out to the world as their image of themselves. This is more a case of a disconnect from the world rather than a closer connection to it.

◇◇◇◇◇◇◇◇

# 25 FEBRUARY 2017
## *Something new I have just learnt*
## *about the Small Intestine*

A patient whose guardian element is Inner Fire (Small Intestine) delighted me this week when she said, rather sadly, 'I run on my thoughts. Other people seem to run on their emotions.'

Cars run on petrol, lorries on diesel, and she recognizes that she 'runs on thoughts'.

Yes, I thought to myself, that is an excellent description of what powers the Small Intestine. It always has to think everything through, sorting and sorting its thoughts out to make sure that its companion official, the Heart, receives good advice. I have described the Small Intestine official as acting as the Heart's secretary, often doing its deep thinking for it, and then passing on what it hopes are only pure thoughts to the master of all, the Heart.

This is how I have learnt to distinguish Inner from Outer Fire, which is never an easy distinction to make. If you think a patient is Fire, ask them some rather complicated question, and watch how they try to answer it. Inner Fire often looks slightly puzzled, frowning a little as it tries first to take in what you are asking, and then start sorting out its reply to your question. There will always be signs of a kind of slight hesitation, as if the answer is not easy to find, and the reply may sound slightly confusing, as though the patient is still sorting out what to say as they talk.

Outer Fire, on the other hand, will tend to give a more straightforward answer, and one which is much less involved in its own thought processes.

Being an Inner Fire person myself, I have often said that I sort my thoughts out as I talk. And now, hearing what my patient said, I agree that I, too, run on my thoughts.

◇◇◇◇◇◇◇◇◇

# 2 MARCH 2107
## *The effect of clearing a CV/GV (Ren Mai/Du Mai) block*

I love hearing patients' descriptions of how specific treatments make them feel. Here is a lovely testimonial to the power of clearing a CV/GV block:

> I feel that this experience has allowed the real essence of who I am to emerge. For the first time in my life I feel that the real me has arrived.

I don't think you can have a more powerful statement explaining the effect of removing this major block to the healthy flow of the elements.

◇◇◇◇◇◇◇◇◇

# 13 MARCH 2017
## *Oh dear! Oh dear! I find that I am addicted!*

I am reading a fascinating book by Adam Alter, *Irresistible: Why We Can't Stop Checking, Scrolling, Clicking and Watching*, about our obsession with our smartphones, our emails, our endless Twitter twittering and our fascination with YouTube.

It makes for a sobering read, none more so than when we are told that leaving a very young child unsupervised in front of those children's gadgets which transfix a child's eyes for hours, but deprive it all too quickly of the ability to look people in the eye, actually damages their little brains. Even something as harmless as talking to a child on Skype reduces the importance of eye-to-eye contact because the child cannot apparently pitch its eyes at the right level on the screen to evoke the kind of immediate response it looks for in the presence of another person.

Not being a two-year-old, why did I come to the depressing conclusion that I, too, was addicted, but what to? Of course, it is to my emails, the only bit of electronic equipment I use. I have, reluctantly, accepted the need for a Facebook account to pass on my blogs to a wider audience; I can go for days without looking at it. But I am, I now realize, hooked on checking to see if any new emails have arrived, so worried I apparently am with the need to answer them immediately, as though not doing so is impolite.

From reading Alter's book, I gather that this is a definite sign of an addiction. I don't have a smartphone so I can only check up on my emails when I am physically sitting in front of my computer, ready to tap away on a large keyboard with an old-fashioned mouse to hand. Having now counted up how often I find myself returning to the computer when I am at home, and realizing that my first action on coming back home is always to hurry to turn it back on again, I acknowledge that I do have as much a problem as if I had immediately to grab a glass of wine if I was a heavy drinker. It may not be as harmful to my health as drinking too much, but it is probably as harmful to my peace of mind in its own way, because each email demands something of me, and often these demands are worrying or disturbing. I am as much in thrall to this wretchedly addictive piece of equipment as anyone hooked to chatting endlessly on Twitter.

Of course, it is not only me, but all those countless others I see in the street or in cafés, their fingers twitching away at their smartphones, their eyes unable to look away to see the world around them, so busy are they scrolling up and down looking for God knows what.

I know that those emailing me can wait a few more hours or even a few more days for an answer from me, so I am resolved to watch myself now and reduce those compulsive excursions of mine to sit in front of the computer. Let's see whether I can manage this!

◇◇◇◇◇◇◇◇

# 14 MARCH 2017
## *Article for the Chinese Culture Research Society of Singapore*

Below is an article about five element acupuncture which an acupuncturist who comes to my seminars in China has asked me to write. I am happy to include it in my blog, as it provides a very general overview of my thinking about five element acupuncture.

### What is five element acupuncture?

Five element acupuncture is a branch of traditional acupuncture which is based on an understanding of the five elements contained in the Nei Jing and handed down over the centuries. It recognizes that the five elements shape each human being, putting the stamp of one of them in particular on each of us. I call this the guardian element. It also goes by the name of the constitutional element. I see it as protecting us when we are in balance, but can cause imbalance when it is under stress from some physical illness or emotional disturbance.

This element is regarded as the dominant element out of the five. It dictates how we look, giving us a colour on our skin (not a racial colour), how we talk, giving us the sound of our voice, how we smell, giving our skin a certain smell, and the emotion which rules our life, such as joy or anger. All these qualities of the elements are those listed in the Nei Jing and are still relevant today. In five element acupuncture, they are used diagnostically to help us treat a patient and restore them to health.

A five element diagnosis is therefore based on what our senses can perceive: the patient's colour, smell, sound of voice and emotion. Students spend a great deal of time developing these skills by training their senses. We know that babies are born with very sensitive senses, but as we grow older we lose much of this sensitivity because we do not practise using our senses. Some of these senses therefore become less acute over time through lack of use, and we forget to pay attention to what they are telling us. We put perfume on our bodies to hide our natural smell, and put make-up on to hide our natural skin colour. Some people can, however, continue to develop very great sensitivity to one sense or another. For example, I have a nearly blind patient who tells me that she knows by a person's smell whether that person is friendly to her or not. A singing teacher will obviously have a highly developed appreciation of the quality of a person's voice.

We obviously use our emotions every day, but because we are social creatures and have had to learn to live among many other people with their own needs and desires, we have learnt to suppress many of our natural emotional responses. Society is also uncomfortable if emotions are expressed too openly.

For example, children are often told by their parents to be friendly and kind to other children, and they soon learn to be careful to suppress their natural anger, and not hit another child if it takes their toys. In fact, children are often told not to express any emotion too strongly. This means that some of these emotions are not allowed their natural outlet, and are forced to stay hidden inside us.

Some of this suppression of our emotions is a natural result of having to live in harmony with our fellow human beings, but if emotions are suppressed too much or for too long they can put great pressure upon us, and in particular upon the guardian element. And this is where the five element acupuncturist, trained to observe changes in the sensory signals from the patient, will assess how far what he/she observes reflects a particular element in balance or out of balance. These changes can be very subtle to start with. That is why a five element practitioner takes time getting to know their patients, asking them about all the stresses in their life, both in the past and in the present, and through this questioning tries to work out which element of the five is the dominant element.

The understanding in five element acupuncture is that it is weaknesses in this element which lead to the appearance of physical and emotional problems. Treatment directed at strengthening the element will give renewed strength and balance, and help the patient deal with the stresses which have led to imbalance. We therefore place great importance on the relationship between the patient and the practitioner, because it is by establishing a good relationship that the patient will feel safe enough with us to take off the social mask we all have to put on in our everyday lives, and show the real nature of who they are and what their problems really are. And it is by allowing the patient to relax with us that the guardian element shows itself most clearly. Then the practitioner can judge from the sensory signals which this element is sending out what treatment the patient needs. For example, a Fire patient's face may be too red, or a Metal patient may appear to be excessively sad.

Treatment is always focused on strengthening the guardian element. It takes time, however, to confirm whether the element we have chosen is the correct one. It is only by assessing the results of treatment, particularly patients' own judgement as to whether their emotional and physical health is improving, that the practitioner can be sure that the diagnosis is correct. It therefore takes courage to be a five element acupuncturist, because no textbook can tell you which element you need to treat. The important thing I always tell students is 'Don't hurry. Don't worry.' Practitioners need to give themselves time to make the correct diagnosis.

Anybody interested in learning more about five element acupuncture will find it helpful to read my *Simple Guide to Five Element Acupuncture* and my *Handbook of Five Element Practice*, both of which books are now available in a Chinese edition. My other three books are available only in English, but are being translated at the moment, and will soon also be published in China.

My great acupuncture master, Professor JR Worsley, always told us that everybody should study the elements, and start to learn to recognize them in all the people around them. Understanding the different qualities of the elements helps us become more tolerant of each other, and makes the world a happier place. For me it is one of the delights of being a five element practitioner that I can help people to a greater understanding of others, and thus make their lives and the lives of their family members and friends more contented.

◇◇◇◇◇◇◇◇

# 23 MARCH 2017
## *Discovering a little gem of a cake shop tucked away behind Oxford Street*

One of the delights of London is how many coffee shops there are, and how often I have managed to find a new one. As everybody who reads my blog knows, it is in coffee shops that I do most of my writing. To think my thoughts, I need the peace of being in my own little world, with no distractions of phone or email to disturb me. If the music is too loud, which unfortunately it often is now, one of the benefits of being hard of hearing and having to wear hearing aids is that at a turn of a little switch I can shut all sound away and stay cocooned in blissful silence for as long as I want.

So today I found yet another little coffee shop, or more correctly a little cake shop. It is called The Sicilian Collection, and is at 51–51A Cleveland Street, London W1T 4JH, email: info@strazzanti.co.

It is run by a young Sicilian woman, Emilia Strazzanti, who has been trained in cake-making by a five-star Michelin chef. Her beautiful cakes are certainly proof of that. I have rarely tasted cakes which are so light to the palette, rich in taste and utterly fresh.

At the moment, the shop is tiny, with just room for a couple of people to sit inside and drink her delicious, freshly made coffee and eat a slice of her cake, and with a bench outside for when the weather gets warmer. She told me, however, that she will soon be extending the shop to the back of the premises, where there will be tables for lunch as well as coffee and cake.

After enjoying two cups of excellent coffee with a slice of one of her cakes, I asked for a selection of three different cakes to take away as a treat for myself. Emilia told me they were slices of:

1. a Sicilian hazelnut and chocolate cake, made from hazelnuts from the north of Catania

2. a Sicilian pistachio and lemon cake with crema di pistachio from Bronte

3. a Sicilian almond cake with almonds from Val di Noto.

I left her little shop with a smile on my face.

# CONCLUSION

This compendium of my blogs came to a natural full-stop with my last blog, *Discovering a little gem of a cake shop tucked away behind Oxford Street*. It so happened that I had nearly finished drawing together all the blogs for this book when I found myself walking past this little café. 'What nicer way to finish this book can there be,' I thought, 'than by writing about one of my great delights, discovering little coffee shops to write in and eating lovely cake?' It seems a cheerful and optimistic way to finish this book in the face of everything else going on in the world at the moment, with Trump in the States and the disaster of Brexit looming over us here. I need to think of things which lighten my heart, and I hope my readers agree.

**Nora Franglen's** own experience of five element acupuncture led her to study at the College of Traditional Acupuncture, Leamington Spa, UK, and she continued her postgraduate studies there under JR Worsley. She was Founder/Principal of the School of Five Element Acupuncture (SOFEA) in London from 1995 to 2007 and continues her teaching through her practice, through postgraduate work in the UK, Europe and China, and now through her successful blog, norafranglen. blogspot.com. Nora is the author of *The Simple Guide to Five Element Acupuncture, The Handbook of Five Element Practice, Patterns of Practice, Keepers of the Soul and On Being a Five Element Acupuncturist*, all also published by Singing Dragon. She lives in London, UK.